PRAISE FOR DR. GUPTE

"The ongoing and significant influences of our conscious and subconscious minds on our everyday health and wellbeing are indisputable. In many ways, our bodies are now understood to be in part reflections of the influences of our minds and emotions. While there are many forms of meditation, such as mindfulness, to help us to purposefully work with our conscious mind and emotions to improve our health and wellbeing, there have been far fewer techniques available to help us similarly harness the workings of our subconscious mind. Dr. Sonia Gupte's work with Integrated Clinical Hypnotherapy addresses this vital need, as it works simultaneously with the conscious and subconscious minds and the body as a whole to achieve enduring healing and transformation. The diverse cases reviewed in this book attest to its ability to treat many illnesses and help individuals live a fruitful and meaningful life."

- Paul J. Mills

Professor and Chief, Family Medicine and Public Health, University of California, San Diego

“Over the past 25 years, as a Head and Neck Cancer Surgeon I have seen tremendous progress made in diagnostic and treatment modalities for this dreadful disease. In the U.S alone more than 16.9 million people are alive today after being diagnosed with Cancer. These survivors deal with a multitude of problems that are difficult to alleviate through traditional methods. Hypnotherapy fills a significant void by helping our patients overcome these physical and emotional hardships. Additionally it can play an important role in smoking cessation and prevention of second cancers. Dr. Gupte has brought a unique, effective and much-needed resource to our survivorship clinics.”

Cherie-Ann Nathan, MD, FACS
Jack Pou Endowed Prof. & Chairman,
Dept. of Otolaryngology/HNS, LSU Health-SHV,
Director of Head and Neck Surgical Oncology,
Feist-Weiller Cancer Center

“Dr. Gupte's unique skill in clinical hypnosis makes readers feel that anything is possible! She blends her artistry in the medical profession with her mastery of language and provides her patients with the innate power to heal themselves. She weaves us through her own personal journey as a healer and a doctor which showcases her true grit to be amongst the few to carve her own path. She teaches us that our limiting beliefs hold us back and once we crack the internal code, we can unleash the person we are meant to be - a beautiful soul with unlimited happiness. Dr. Gupte has already changed the medical profession for the better and she demonstrates through her patients that hypnotherapy is one of the most efficacious modalities 'modern' medicine has to offer."

- Rupa Mahadevan, MD, FAAP, ABOIM

"Sonia is an effective and skilled hypnotherapist. She is also a superb speaker and presents her insights relating to the hypnotic trance and it's therapeutic effects so eloquently. She is a passionate, talented medical practitioner and hypnotherapist. This unique combination harnesses a depth of medical knowledge coupled with the power of the hypnotic trance to effect lasting change at the subconscious level of all those who seek her. In her book Sonia showcases not only her own talent and expertise but the exceptional effects of hypnosis in freeing the body, mind and soul of debilitating and limiting beliefs. Her work is exemplary and absolutely needed during these times of great change in our human psyche. Congratulations to Sonia for this epic and timely book!"

- Chiara Marrapodi
Director of Lifelong Learning
California Institute for Human Science

"Working with Sonia was truly a life-changing experience. Everything shifted for the better. I was just so amazed at the speed of how things happened and the clarity I received. I highly recommend working with Sonia if you feel stuck in any area of your life."

- E.S.

"Thank you for giving me my son back. He hasn't had a night terror since his sessions and sleeps so deeply. He is much easier to be around now and there is lots more laughter in our family. He is more confident, too. Thank you from the bottom of my heart for all you have done for him."

- C.D.

"During my sessions, I realized that I was holding onto emotions of the past which were making me physically sick. After the session, I started feeling so much better. Hypnotherapy was a blessing for me!"

- N.T.

"I suffered from peripheral neuropathy that badly affected the left side of my body. It was so severe, I was in pain from the top of my head to the tip of my little toe. After a trip to the ER, I only felt 10% better. After one session with Dr. Sonia I felt a 50% shift in my pain and have been on the path to recovery ever since. Without this session, my healing might have taken months. Thank you Dr. Sonia for being my angel."

- A.N.

"I have fought emotional eating and my weight for most of my adult life. I tried medications, herbal and naturopathic remedies and changed my diet with no result. Then I met Dr. Sonia. Since our sessions I don't recognize the person I've become. I've lost 10 pounds!"

- C.K.

Dear Patti,

Happy reading!

WITHIN

Love

Sonia :)

April '24

WITHIN

Finding Yourself, Fixing What's Broken,
& Finally Reclaiming True Health

DR. SONIA GUPTE

with

JULIE TRAGER, MSW

HOLLAND HOUSE
PUBLISHING

NEW YORK

WITHIN : Finding Yourself, Fixing What's Broken,
& Finally Reclaiming True Health

For information contact:
HollandHousePublishing.com

ISBN: 978-0-578-72946-6
First Edition: January 2021

10 9 8 7 6 5 4 3 2 1

TABLE OF CONTENTS

ACKNOWLEDGEMENTS

As the saying goes: "Behind every successful Man there is a Woman." In my case it fits the opposite way! I would like to acknowledge and thank a few very special men in my life who have nurtured me, guided me, and made me who I am today. It's because of their support that I'm able to stand tall and proud as a successful woman.

First my father, who loved me unconditionally and instilled a confidence which remains unshaken to this day. He always believes in me and supports the choices and decisions I make as I explore life under his guidance.

I remember a time when, as a young doctor, I had to use public transport to reach the hospital during the odd hours of the day. On one such evening, a rusted nail ripped through my pants as I was getting off the bus. I was furious by the time I reached the hospital, desperately trying to hide my torn clothing. When I reached home after work, I was still fuming. I told my father what had happened and declared that I would no longer ride on public transit. I wanted my own car. I belonged to an upper middle-class family, and though I was not brought up as a spoiled brat, there is no memory I have where a legitimate desire of mine was not fulfilled by my beloved father. And true to style, within a week, I had a car... brand new, the latest model! I was thrilled; and even though I was a newbie at driving, my dad never doubted my ability to drive independently. But within a week, while reversing out of a tight alley, I collided with a pillar. The door on the passenger side was a complete wreck. With a grim, sad face I came home and told dad that the car had been damaged and I will never forget his reaction. Instead of being angry, he simply asked: "*Are you okay*?" I know it cost him a fortune to get the damage fixed - the entire door had to be replaced - yet he never mentioned it. Not once. When I got the car back, fully repaired and looking brand new, he simply gave me the keys and told me to drive safe! I excelled in driving after that, as no one had created doubts in my mind or made me feel guilty. I understood where I was lacking and simply took up the challenge to master my weaknesses. This is just one example of my father being that very first pillar who enabled me to stand tall, on my own two feet. Through his unending support, he is the one who showed me what I am truly capable of.

I love you more than anything Papaji. Thank you for making me who I am today!

Next, I wish to acknowledge my beloved husband, Jit. Being in the institution of marriage for nearly two decades now has been such an exciting journey. From meeting him online as a stranger, to becoming a spouse in a short period of four months and moving to an entirely new country... looking back, it seems almost like a dream! In addition to being a loving and affectionate husband, Jit took up the role of mentor. When I moved with him to Singapore, I was in the very early stages of my medical career and obviously had high ambitions; but these dreams came crashing down when my application for a practicing license was rejected by the Singapore Medical Council due to my Russian medical degree. I was confused and almost depressed, sensing my medical career had finished even before it started. But Jit shifted into gear and inspired me to not give up. He told me that we were going to fight to make my dreams a reality, and that's exactly what we did. We filed an appeal for reconsideration. After eight months of hard work and perseverance, I was the first ever doctor with a Russian medical degree to get a license to practice in Singapore! It was an incredible feat and served as a solid foundation, not only for our relationship but my medical career. Through this experience I got a chance to learn and gain experience at world-class teaching hospitals in Singapore. I have always looked to Jit for guidance in moments of doubt. Our relationship continues to evolve and thrive as we move from one milestone to the next. He has always encouraged me and taken pride in my accomplishments.

Jit, thank you for being the wind beneath my wings, for making me feel that the sky is the limit and that I can accomplish any goal I set my sights on. I love you more than words can express!

My next big thanks go to my two beautiful boys, Tanay and Taran, who make me a proud mother every day and enable me to feel the blessings of being unconditionally loved!

Thank you Tanu for being calm and composed while handling your tyrannous little brother with such patience, and for lending a helping hand whenever mom needs one. I am so proud of you for the man you are becoming. Thank you Taru for your unlimited hugs and kisses. You give me invincible power and energy! You are my sunshine!

The last very special person I wish to acknowledge is my mentor, my guru, Yuvraj Kapadia. I have such tremendous gratitude for you! Yuvraj is the founder of EKAA Clinical Hypnotherapy Foundation and the mastermind behind this very unique hypnotherapy training program. EKAA integrates ancient esoteric wisdom and western clinical practices to offer the most innovative and comprehensive hypnotherapy certification in the world. This book showcases the hypnotherapy skills I have acquired through training that is unparalleled in its depth and has the power to truly transform life. "*Heal while you learn and learn while you heal*" is EKAA's mantra! Yuvraj, the passion I have for hypnotherapy has grown deep roots because of you.

My first meeting with Yuvraj was seven years ago at the writing of this book, but it is still so fresh in my mind. I bumped into him in an elevator during my lunch break while I was studying hypnotherapy in the same facility where he was teaching another group. I was in awe at meeting the founder of the course, and we got to talking. He asked me about my thoughts on the course and I told him that at that point in time I was skeptical, but curious; and that I wanted to delve deeper into the modality. He replied that he had trained thousands of students globally, many of whom are medical professionals and doctors, who had already become facilitators and went on to train others as well. In that moment I couldn't help but wonder what kind of doctor would choose to train hypnotherapists over their medical practice. Yet not seven years later and I, too, have become one of those doctors!

Yuvraj, thank you for always watching over my back, for being my teacher and grounding me when I feel I am losing hope. Most of all, thank you for believing in my passion and my purpose!

FOREWORD

To all of you who have just picked up this book and have begun browsing through it, I would suggest... take a few deep breaths before you proceed any further. Deep breaths, just so that you are prepared in an astounding, mind-boggling way to receive what this compilation is going to unleash on you.

Health, as a derivative of "heal" (which in turn draws its essence from the ancient language reference of *hale* - a word meant to imply strength, return to wholesomeness, free from ailment, a restoration of a complete state) is a term that exists at the very fulcrum of human existence. All our accomplishments and advancements as a human race have been hugely dependant on a factor that we sometimes take for granted - that of our health.

So, the million-dollar question is: What makes us as humans wholesome and complete? Is it just our physical machinery that we call a body? What good would a body be if it is stressed with fear or obsessed with anger? And to say nothing of a terrible, drained energetic state where waking up every morning is simply the worst drudgery that one could get enmeshed in? Conversely, simply having a happy disposition is not enough for us to function at peak potential if our body is racked with disease and disorder.

It is high time that, as an intelligent and constantly evolving species, we wake up to and embrace the paradigm of integral health. We now, more than ever, require rewriting of our clichéd understanding of health.

For us to be able to explore and live out our life to its highest potential, we must not only maintain our HARDWARE of the human computer that we call THE BODY, but we must also ensure, beyond doubt, that this hardware is suitably formatted to be able to permit A VIRUS-FREE SOFTWARE PROGRAM, that we call the MIND, to effectively function, using it adroitly and smartly.

Having personally grown up in a family of medical professionals, I was naturally attuned to the medical model of human healthcare. Yet, with time and the vagaries of life, I concluded that though our technological advancement in terms of managing and improving physical health was speeding ahead, our "software" understanding and servicing stayed stuck in the archaic traditional approach of mental disease.

A fresh amalgamation of understanding the mind as the invisible body (or viewing the body as the visible mind) emerged in my awareness as a much-needed perception changer. And Dr. Sonia Gupte walked into my curriculum as an indication from the Universe.

From being a curious medical graduate who seemed to have developed a fancy for the new age healing movement, to a very focused and committed professional who is now tirelessly working to this game-changing blend, Dr. Sonia has indeed come a long way.

With a sedate start as an adroit and curious student, to an excited hypnotherapy intern, and then from a flourishing medical doctor to a path-breaking hypnotherapist who now teaches the EKAA hypnotherapy curriculum, Dr. Sonia Gupte seems to have found the plethora of resources needed that will be required to effect this monumental change in human healthcare. Her vision is a direct answer to my musings and seems to convince me that what seemed like a distant pipedream a few years ago can indeed become our empowered healthcare reality.

Her book is a testimonial not only to her beliefs but also an offering to all of us who view the Human system as a living, thinking, feeling, and intelligent being that requires a broader spectrum of focus, bringing together the best of the physical and ethereal approach to wellbeing and healthcare.

Happy Reading!

Yuvraj Kapadia

Founder & CEO

EKAA Integrated Clinical Hypnotherapy Foundation

PREFACE

"I am a woman, a doctor, a wife,
a mother, a sister, the child of a fiery father,
a big-picture thinker and a traveler on the
road of the shero's journey.
All of these parts of me came together
in this book. Thank you for walking
a little of my path with me."

I have long known that being a doctor is my true calling, but after fifteen years in practice, I felt a little unfulfilled. Somehow I sensed that I was vaguely *incomplete*. It wasn't until my mom tried to commit suicide that this feeling crystalized into something more concrete. This experience forever changed me. It shook me to my core. Suddenly, I was ignited with this need to search, though I had no idea what I was searching for. In hindsight, that need was connected to a very specific void. *I was a doctor who was missing the healer within.*

I got into healthcare because I care deeply about others and have a tremendous desire to see those I serve live healthy, fulfilling, amazing lives. But the day-to-day world of medicine that deals with the typical ills of the human body isn't fairing so well. In my practice, I had patients who clearly felt unwell - yet when I ran labs and other diagnostics, the results came back normal. When I told these patients that I could find nothing conclusive, they would look at me with those eyes and say, "*But Doctor, I KNOW there is something wrong with me!*"

There were more times than I care to admit in these situations when I was tapped out in terms of a solution. I could write them a prescription to manage their symptoms; the medications would make them feel a little better (but not for long); and then they would come back for a refill... month after month. At the same time, I saw medications fail in a very personal way, both when my mom attempted suicide, despite being on a number of anti-depressant prescriptions; and when my dad continued to functionally decline, despite medications and surgical intervention for his cervical myelopathy.

I am so proud of my profession. I know without a doubt that doctors and the modern medical system can be the stars in an otherwise dark sky. In the midst of COVID-19, healthcare providers can be seen working with superhero-like stamina to take care of unbelievably sick patients, pivoting constantly to dart around the barriers of ever-changing demands, risking their own safety and that of their families to save the lives of perfect strangers. But despite our brilliance when it comes to critical care, I believe there is something inherent in the way we practice medicine that needs attention. I know it is unfashionable to say, but when it comes to chronic disease, we participate in a system that leaves everyone wanting. If only we could better manage chronic disease by reducing dependency on medications and diminishing the impact of chronic disease on the body, would pandemics like COVID-19 have a different outcome?

As a doctor, my overwhelming desire was to cure, but it felt like I was just treating symptoms, never knowing or reaching the cause. This restlessness made me ask some key questions. "*What if I had different tools in my toolbox as a physician? What if I stopped thinking that my medical training taught me everything I needed to know? What if I accepted that modern medicine is missing a critical ingredient?*" Spending time with these questions changed everything for me.

I wrote this book because, particularly in the wake of COVID-19, I believe it is more important than ever to treat chronic disease differently. Less chronic disease means more survivors in the wake of another pandemic, more patients living their best lives, and more doctors benefitting from the joy of truly being a healer. We all want that. It's why we are here and why we work so hard.

I've witnessed what seem like miracles using hypnotherapy, but really, it's just evidence that working with both mind and body simultaneously can achieve results superior to working with the physiology alone. This book is my way of sharing that evidence with you.

By chronicling some of my favorite cases that highlight the interplay between mind and body, emotion and life experience, disease and health, I will shine a light on our ability to completely revolutionize modern medicine.

"I have hung up my stethoscope
to pursue a different way of healing -
and that is what I intend to
share with this book."

This book is my "love letter" to the amazing modality of hypnotherapy!

Dr. Sonia Gupte

Founder & CEO

Enso-nia Center for Mind and Life Transformation

San Diego, California

INTRODUCTION

"Can Our Thoughts Create a Disease?"

The mind is a powerful tool for healing. This concept is not only shockingly underutilized in modern medicine; it is scoffed at and derided. But research has shown that the mind generates 50,000 to 60,000 thoughts a day. It's like a computer that generates data nonstop - and in the world of the body, that data can have a significant impact on your physiology. As an example, close your eyes and think of an evening in your life when everything was perfect: the company, the setting, the conversation, the feeling of camaraderie, the wine, the food. As you see that night playing out in your mind's eye, feel what happens in your body. Notice that the muscles in your shoulders relax, that tension you carry in your stomach subsides, your jaw relaxes. Maybe you start to smile. Recognize that the thought of the past generated a relaxation response and an emotion of happiness. Now flip it. Close your eyes again and think of an argument you had with a boss or your spouse, or even the news that you watched last night. Now how do you feel?

What sensations and emotions are generated by these less positive memories? What body sensations come up? Where do you feel tense?

So, in any situation, thoughts continuously originate in our mind. These thoughts can be associated with memories from our past. And because of this association, certain thoughts organically generate an emotion. The Latin derivative for the word emotion, *emotere*, literally means "energy in motion." This emotional energy creates a sensation, a physiological reaction, which is felt in the body. Generally, the energy of a positive or happy emotion is felt and eventually released. However, if it is an emotion coming from an unpleasant or traumatic event, we are usually unable to digest or process it. Undigested or suppressed emotional energy tends to remain stuck somewhere within our body. As time goes by, we consciously forget about that event, but the memory of that event remains stored in our subconscious mind. That forgotten or suppressed memory with the undigested emotion keeps circulating like an invisible live wire connecting the mind with the body. In the present, seemingly inconsequential, everyday events can trigger that same undigested emotion until one day, many triggers later, the body is unable to handle it and you could be diagnosed with a "Dis-ease." This process of "thoughts causing a Dis-ease" can unfold in as little as six months!

THOUGHT-E~MOTION-ENERGY - BODY - *"DIS-EASE"*

"When one gets diagnosed with a 'Dis-ease' it's a clear indication that the physical body is trying to showcase the suppressed and ignored side of the Mind!"

Do you know anyone with back pain that has no apparent causation and is not amenable to physiotherapy, chiropractic, or other treatments? Or someone with persistent intestinal pain so severe that they've been hospitalized, but whose scans repeatedly come up negative? Since our current state of western medicine fails to come up with a treatment that works, could we consider that may be the cause is actually buried in the mind, leading to the "Dis-ease"?

Many times I am asked to explain the difference between the *brain* and the *mind*. To keep it simple, imagine the brain as the *hardware* and the mind as the *software* of your body's computer. Research has confirmed that we only use about 10% of our mind, defined as our conscious ability to logically analyze and think; the other 90% is the automated processes of our subconscious or unconscious. Continuing the analogy of a computer, the subconscious is like the *hard disk* while the conscious mind is the *CPU*. From the moment you were born, your subconscious mind has collected zillions of memories and embedded them on a hard disk that, as it turns out, isn't so easy to access.

Science has also found that the subconscious zone is much more powerful than the logical, conscious side - which is why we keep doing the same things over and over again, even though it does not make logical sense. We keep making the same mistakes, falling back into the same addictions, or the same relationships, even if they are painful and lead to unhappiness and poor health. Have you ever wondered why we are unable to break out of these patterns? It's because (unbeknownst to your conscious mind) the subconscious takes over, almost like a very powerful photocopying machine, duplicating whatever we store within. And those traumatic memories from the past, tainted with the undischarged emotions, creates a "corrupted file" that hijacks the logical operation of the mind.

Knowing that your subconscious is almost 6,000 times more powerful than the logical, thinking, conscious mind, it opens up a whole new rationale as to why certain self-sabotaging thoughts, behaviors, *even ailments,* often have no logical premise - and yet the pain and suffering they cause is undeniable.

They say "*time heals*" but that's often not true - specifically in the case of traumatic or difficult situations we have faced in the past.

More so when we are young, have fewer coping skills, and possess a limited understanding of the world. Those traumatic memories from our past tainted, with our undigested emotions, creates what I call a "corrupted file" in our subconscious mind.

So the elementary school kid who was repeatedly bullied; or the ten-year-old who overheard his parents talking about filing for bankruptcy; or the five-year-old who was sexually abused by a family member (and no one believed her); they all subconsciously hold unexpressed emotions from the past that can create a "corrupted file." Whether it's anger, sadness, fear, or helplessness - the primary core emotions that cause an energetic burden if not dealt with - this suppression can wreak havoc on the body in the long run.

"It is these past memories with undigested emotions which end up creating issues in the present that don't seem to have much basis in reality."

So how do we deal with these corrupted files? The best way I've found is through hypnotherapy. For clarity, *hypnotherapy* is *therapy done in the state of hypnosis*. What is hypnosis? It is the physically and mentally relaxed state in which we can access the otherwise hard-to-get information coded in the subconscious mind. We experience mild forms of hypnosis daily. Have you ever driven to the grocery and couldn't remember how you got there because your mind was "somewhere else"? Have you ever heard an old song that took you back to the *exact* time and place when you first heard it twenty years ago? These are all mild forms of self-hypnosis. The difference between this and guided hypnotherapy is that the hypnotherapist *guides* the client to enter his subconscious in a relaxed state. In that relaxed state the client is guided to travel back in time to a specific childhood memory. Once at the nexus of that memory, the wisdom of the present-day adult helps his younger self digest the situation of the past - that unhealed, traumatic emotion - from a new perspective to find closure. All of this happens in the safety of the person's mind, being skillfully navigated by the hypnotherapist. The miracle is that as you reach out to your younger self and heal that past situation in the subconscious, you also heal its current manifestation of "Dis-ease" in the present.

"And in the process, you become your own savior!"

The job of a good hypnotherapist is simply to help their client access the stored memories, retrieve the corrupted files, and rescript the unwanted data while leaving the memory intact.

As a hypnotherapist, I have witnessed transformation of complex physical and psychological issues that I know I would not have resolved as a physician. I have helped patients with gastritis, GERD, IBS, obesity, smoking addiction, anxiety, depression, phobias, pain, and countless other conditions. I consistently hear client after client tell me –

"I've done so many things to make this problem better. Now I understand why all of those things didn't work."

Initially, I integrated hypnotherapy with my mainstream practice, offering my patients the typical western treatment with hypnotherapy sessions as an alternative. Because of my success, it didn't take me long to leave my traditional practice for good, choosing to use hypnotherapy alone to treat those who come to me – often, after having worked with family doctors, specialists, therapists, and psychiatrists but found no real improvement in their condition. The profound changes I have seen are beautiful and give credence to the intimate connection between mind and body. Hypnotherapy can heal when dealing solely with the physiology cannot.

The mind is often the key to anything that is not working well in your life. It is my hope that after reading this book you will start to understand the need to embrace Mind/Body medicine through hypnotherapy. It's my firm belief that integrating this modality into medical practice will not only transform patients' lives, but physicians' lives, too. It most definitely renewed my love for my calling! *I am now an expanded, more joyful version of my former self.*

In this book, you will find a bigger discussion of the limitations of treating patients purely as physical bodies, and a review of the history of hypnosis in medicine. You will hear more of my personal story, and my journey so far, having found my purpose with this modality. Most importantly, I will share a variety of cases so you can get a bird's-eye view of my process and some of the major transformations in the health of my patients.

Each patient case is divided into three separate sections: *The Problem* - the issues they presented in their intake; *The Sessions* - a description of the way each patient was navigated in their hypnotherapy session to achieve healing; and *The Outcome* - which describes my take on the case as a Physician.

As a side note, I don't go into details regarding my process of bringing people into the hypnotic state because it's so similar each time; just know that each session begins with the patient already relaxed and deeply in their subconscious.

What you won't see much in this book are references, links to studies, footnotes or citations. At first, I went the route of making this information of more academic relevance; I quickly changed course as the chapters started to look like a medical journal - dry and devoid of emotions - which did not fulfill my two major reasons for writing this book.

My first intention is that this book will expand your mind beyond the science that is most often in front of you. Hypnotherapy studies and results are definitely out there; yet, if I have discovered anything, it's that the randomized controlled trial can't be the be-all, end-all of our scientific exploration into health and healing. We are dealing with complex, unique human beings that can't be compartmentalized, sectioned-off, or sanitized. I have achieved amazing results with hundreds of patients, and some of those cases are presented in this book as my own way of showcasing evidence. I hope you will agree, after reading these case studies, that we must be more open as a society to other forms of scientific rigor. It is now deeply ingrained in me that when we are working with people, our acknowledgment of their uniqueness must be part of the equation.

Second, I want you to really connect with my brave and beautiful patients: to go with me on the ride of each hypnotherapy session without thinking too much. I want you to immerse yourself in the experience, because at the end of the day, for me it's that connection that matters the most. Hypnotherapy has brought me back to the heart of healing; and I hope in some small way that reading about their intimate journeys (and mine) will do this for you, too.

In fact, I've written this book for both physicians and patients. For that reason, the writing is clear, easy-to-understand, and mostly free from medical jargon. I know that there is an ever-increasing number of doctors and patients who have become frustrated with the limitations of modern medicine and want to go deeper to find alternatives that have a higher level of success. These cases are meant for those who are bold enough to consider options outside of the traditional paradigm.

It is my hope that, together, we will choose to usher in a much-needed shift in modern medicine, one that surpasses that of the cookie-cutter, one-protocol-fits-all system we now have, in order to embrace the singular, wonderful creatures we all are.

"True health is not just about living disease-free. It's the best prescription for all of us to live energetic, productive, joyful, amazing lives."

"WHEN WE DARE TO DO SOMETHING DIFFERENT, WE CAN LITERALLY CHANGE THE WORLD!"

CHAPTER ONE

LUKE: THE BODY ALWAYS TALKS

"This is what doctors must know."

THE PROBLEM

Luke is a well-built man in his twenties who looks adorably geeky and upon conversation, is a very no-nonsense type of guy. He has suffered from migraines since the age of seven. Since then, he has never had a day without a headache. However, at the time of our meeting, the headaches had become much worse, to the point of blackouts. Now he frequently logs a pain score of 8 out of 10, with a pain score of 10 and beyond not uncommon. These headaches have completely stopped his life. In Luke's own words...

"As a child till teenager, I tried many different headache/migraine medications; however, they didn't help at all. The medications most of the time made it worse or did nothing at all. It was just false hope that it will cure me of my curse. I had a neurologist check me for any abnormality with CT and MRI scans; however, there was nothing but a benign abnormality. In 2017 I enlisted into the military; however, I was discharged... because of my debilitating migraines. I've lost important relationships because of this migraine, so after the military discharge I tried looking for clinical trials. It didn't help. After all that, a buddy of mine suggested I go to a chiropractor. I spent over six months with the chiropractor, yet it was just temporary relief, like seeing a mirage after being stranded in the desert. As I kept trying to find a way to cure this curse I was finally at the end of my rope. I had lost hope."

By the time we start our work together, Luke is desperate. It was his dream as a young boy to join the military, so his medical discharge is devastating. He now lives at home with his family because he is unable to hold down a job. He's undergone extensive testing, both in and out of the military, with no resulting diagnosis. He has tried all of the typical medications for migraine headaches but none of the meds make a dent in his pain. In fact, with most of them, his pain actually gets worse. Because he has blown through all of the diagnostics, prescriptions, and treatments that I would have recommended as a GP, I work with Luke using hypnotherapy to find the original cause of these migraines and the reason they worsened seven years ago.

CHAPTER ONE

THE SESSION

In our only session, I ask Luke once he is under hypnosis, "Now you will become aware of the reason you are having these migraines. Please describe to me how this reason looks or appears to you." After a moment, he sees himself as a boy of six or seven years old. I ask him, "What is the expression on his face?" After a few minutes of silence, I gently ask Luke what is happening and he relates that his younger self is actually hitting him, pounding him with his fists. "He is very upset with me. He is yelling at me, saying 'Where were you? I needed your help! I needed you!!!'"

Your "inner child" is the impression of your own younger self showcasing an unresolved issue from the past. I have never seen an inner child hitting the present adult within a session! Recovering from my surprise, I ask Luke, "*What happened when you were six or seven years old?*" Luke answers, "*I was sexually abused by a close relative, repeatedly. I didn't know who to turn to; I felt no one would believe me. I was helpless, angry and scared.*"

Now I understand that while he attempted to bury those memories from his past, the wounds are still raw. Luke's inner child created the pain of those headaches as if trying to get Luke's attention because he desperately needed to deal with those long-standing emotions that were never processed.

Having understood the reason of this rage, I ask Luke to comfort that younger self. "Let him know that you, as the adult, didn't know how to reach him before but now you are here to protect him."

As the young Luke is soothed, I ask the adult Luke to call in that relative who abused him. "Luke, I want you to keep the child safe with you, and sense the presence of that person who abused you. When you sense that, let me know." Eventually, Luke nodded, "Yes." "How does the child feel when he sees him?" Luke indicates that the child is scared and is hiding behind him. I then ask the adult Luke, "I want you to empower this child by standing beside him, and then tell me what you sense. What would he like to do?" Luke replies, "He wants to hit this man. He wants to hit him hard."

The beauty of hypnotherapy is that, within a safe space created in the mind, this child gets to do to what he could not do then. With the help of his adult self, the child who was powerless is now feeling protected. I instruct Luke, "*Let the child do whatever he wants to do, whatever he needs to do to find closure.*" I stay quiet for some time to let this drama unfold in Luke's subconscious mind, allowing him to release the stuck energies of anger, fear, hatred, and helplessness. I finally ask, "*How does the child feel?*" Luke replies, "*He is thankful, and relieved. He has a new child-like energy.*" I further guide him, "*Now as the adult, find your own closure with this man*. Express whatever you always wished to say to him." This takes a while and then Luke tells me, "*It's done. I kicked him out.*" I ask, "*How is the child now?*" and Luke responds, "*He is looking at me with gratitude and admiration.*"

When Luke opens his eyes, his pain score, which had been a 10 when the session started, is now a 2!! Within a single 90-minute session we have discovered the root of his headaches and reduced his pain score to a level he hasn't experienced in the past seven years. We also got an answer to my main question, which was, "*What caused the migraines to worsen seven years ago*?" After our session ended, Luke told me that it was seven years ago: that was when he found out that his abuser had also molested his younger sister.

When I checked in on him after six months, Luke was taking college classes and working with the military to re-enlist.

In his testimonial, he wrote...

> *"The day before my session, I awoke from a panic attack in the middle of the night. I was afraid that this was just like the others and that there was no future for me. March 2019, my first session with Dr. Sonia, was more helpful than all that money spent on medication and chiropractor sessions. I had finally found a way out of my nightmare. I was able to solve my traumas and fears that were affecting my mind that caused my migraines. As of now, my migraines are not at the pain scale of 7-8 constantly every second anymore, but a mild sporadic one with maybe a 2-4. I don't black out anymore, and I am doing pretty good in school now."*

When I ask how his coursework is going, he says, "*I couldn't think before but now my head is clear. I am doing well.*" Throughout the last year, Luke has come back for three more sessions to further work on himself. Though he has some headaches occasionally, they have never come close to the intensity or frequency he experienced before. His migraines no longer stop him from living his life.

THE OUTCOME

As a doctor, I wouldn't have known how to deal with Luke's trauma; in fact, I likely wouldn't have discovered it. I wasn't trained to look beyond the physical. Like Luke, I've met so many patients who have a chronic illness that doesn't respond to medications, and these cases have shown me that by separating mind and body I'm not able to fully support my patients, especially those who have experienced trauma or have an intractable illness. Now, when someone walks into my office who hasn't gotten better despite taking a lot of meds, I know that it's time to start searching for more than just a physical cause.

When we experience trauma we are typically afraid to revisit it, but Luke taught me that we can be empowered through our vulnerability. Vulnerability is often seen as weakness in our culture, particularly with men and boys; but thinking this way leads not only to disease, but often to a broken life. If we are to remain healthy in body, mind, and spirit we must give ourselves permission - men as well as women, boys as well as girls - to embrace our most difficult experiences without being shamed or ashamed. When we do, we become the strongest version of ourselves. Hypnotherapy equips people to face their vulnerabilities with the benefit of immediate release and catharsis. When this is done well, within the safety and support of the hypnotherapeutic milieu, it is incredibly powerful, beautiful, and completely life-changing.

In Luke's own words, "I don't ever remember feeling like this."

When I began to have the kind of success with other patients that I had achieved with Luke, I began to thoroughly integrate hypnotherapy into my practice. The more I did so, the more I thought, "*This is what doctors must know.*"

"Being able to work with the mind - that's the skill we are lacking that can make all the difference."

FREE RESOURCE

Could you benefit from hypnotherapy if you have a chronic disease? Download this PDF assessment to learn more.

https://www.enso-nia.com/within/resources

CHAPTER TWO

SONIA: BECOMING

"When your whole world is suddenly foreign, you start to look at challenges in a different way."

I am the eldest of three daughters. I am lucky; I grew up with a lot of love. My dad, the unquestionable head of the family, was not only there for my mom, myself, and my siblings, but was also a strong pillar of support for his family of origin that includes eight siblings.

My dad is fierce. He always tells the story of how he started out earning just a handful of rupees and thought, "*Why am I working for someone else when I can do something on my own?*" So, when I was born, he took that leap of faith and left his secure (if not lucrative) job and started his own business. It took time but it was a success! He started out with one small photography shop and ended up with six centers across India. I always used to hear as a child, "*You can do whatever you want to do*." It is his success, his ability to dream and take risks, that gives me my confidence today.

I was in third grade and my sister and I were supposed to go to a brand-new school. Instead of my dad taking us on our first day, he just put on our backpacks and said "*Go*," and we're like, "*You mean, alone*?" With his ever-calm demeanor, he just says, "*Yeah, just go see the teacher and say hello.*" It was a little nerve wracking, but he had this unshakeable confidence in us - so we did it. Looking back now, I feel it was experiences like this that laid the solid foundation on which I proudly stand to this day.

Throughout my early years, I had wanted to be all kinds of things. I wanted to be in the army, then a flight attendant, or a pilot. I wanted to be everything - every year I wanted to do something different. I didn't decide I wanted to be a doctor until the end of high school. The entrance exams for any science-related college-level program are exceptionally competitive in India. Unfortunately, I didn't make it in. But I wanted to be a doctor so badly, I kept looking for another way. That's when I found the medical scholarship in Russia.

I was seventeen when I left home to study medicine. I had only occasionally traveled abroad but never lived alone. The medical curriculum was in the Russian language, and I didn't know the language at all; hence the curriculum required an additional year just to study the language itself. Despite all this, it was super exciting for me to leave India to do something adventurous. There was the excitement of traveling, being on my own, learning a foreign language, and learning how to be a physician - my chosen career and passion.

This was not an easy journey. It gave me a vastly different background compared to most doctors I know. When your *whole world* is suddenly upended - when you have to study, write, and learn something as complex as medicine in a different language while living alone in foreign country - you start to look at challenges in a different way. It gives you this confidence that you can not only handle anything, but also that you can find new ways of dealing with problems. Back then, I was connected to my own power, coming fresh out of my family home and my dad's influence. I'll admit that the passion, the drive, and motivation with which this journey began was somewhere lost a few years back when I sensed that deep void within.

And then hypnotherapy happened to me...

"I have finally found my purpose!

CHAPTER THREE

NIDHI: THE RIPPLE EFFECT

"Why am I never good enough?"

THE PROBLEM

Born and raised in India, Nidhi is filled with sunshine. Her smile is so big she lights up everything around her and she is exceptionally positive. I met her through her sister, who had chronic gastritis for which she was consulting me, and who also had difficulty getting pregnant for some time. When she saw her sister not only feeling physically better but becoming pregnant within a month after our sessions, she felt motivated to try it herself.

Nidhi came to me for weight loss. She had a stubborn forty pounds that just wouldn't come off no matter what she did. In Indian culture, marriage for a woman is still a big deal. If you are in your mid-twenties and haven't been proposed to yet, you will likely get some pressure from your family. Nidhi's parents were introducing her to lots of eligible men, but she wasn't interested in any of them. Both she and her family blamed her lack of marriageability on the weight she had gained since being diagnosed with a hypoactive thyroid a few years back. Even Nidhi wondered if her own disinterest was because she didn't feel any connection to the bachelors, or because she was so self-conscious about her weight that she wouldn't let herself be vulnerable and open to a relationship.

It was doubly hard to be overweight at this point in her life because she had always been thin growing up. She never had to worry about what she ate. Though she did have a thyroid condition, she ate healthy foods, didn't overeat, exercised, and loved being outdoors. She had seen physicians regularly and followed their protocols, including taking her thyroid medication. She told me she had tried everything she could think of.

Nidhi also asked for help with a lifetime of anger and frustration. Over the years, many people in her life had judged her and forced her into things that she knew weren't in her best interest. She was aware that this anger and frustration stemmed from authority figures who had bullied her in a variety of ways and who also failed to appreciate her hard work, intelligence, and fortitude.

While I didn't deny that her thyroid was a factor, I thought I could support her by tapping on the power of the mind to lose weight by working through any stuck emotions that might be hindering her efforts. She was carrying both anger and weight. I wondered: Could there be a connection?

THE SESSIONS

Nidhi vividly remembers her first session because it was incredibly intense. "*I cried so much.*" When she found herself, in trance at the age of seven or eight, playing badminton, climbing trees, just running around - connected with a feeling of being so carefree - she understood that while she loved to be spontaneous and creative as a kid, her mom was very serious about her studies and would try to force her to sit with her books. And Nidhi? Well... she just wanted to be a kid. She wanted to move and run. She wanted to just BE.

This was the start of her anger and frustration - being forced by the authority to follow a structure and to perform according to that structure, instead of just being who she was: a bright, artistic, creative, boisterous kid. Though she tried to make the people in her life happy by suffering through her studies, she remembers the time when she eventually stopped caring about what others wanted her to do. But when she stopped caring, she also shut down. She spent hours hiding away in her room, refusing to communicate with her family, and crying in the bathroom to release pent up emotion. "*I had a lot of those bathroom sessions.*" While she was thin at the time, we discovered in session that this was the true start of pent up emotions that would lead to her weight issues later.

There were so many areas of her life where this judgment, this constant criticism, this trying to get her to conform to structures that didn't suit her, showed up over the next fifteen years. In high school, college, post-college, her first years working as a teacher - and finally, when she couldn't find a suitable mate for marriage. Her conclusions about herself and her life?

"No one understands me."

"They will scold me and judge me."

"Everything is forced on me."

"I must always prove myself."

"I am alone; there is no one to help me."

There was a deep sense of betrayal as family, teachers, friends, and colleagues judged her and failed to support her in one way or another. What Nidhi didn't realize was that her early years had become a self-fulfilling prophecy.

Her body also betrayed her, beginning in her teens. Her pent-up emotions, the continual criticism, lack of support, and lack of understanding began to put wear and tear on her body, leading to a vicious feedback loop of criticism, getting sick, and further criticism. Once again, no one cut her a break; and she used to cry from both pain and total overwhelm. She ultimately developed hypoactive thyroid, which caused her to gain weight just when she wanted to seriously date and marry.

I remember that Nidhi's sessions were filled with releasing of suppressed emotions (*catharsis*). I came to understand that she had a profound sorrow around the fact that she was never allowed to live in a way that was true to herself. In fact, it didn't matter whether she was acting within her own best interests or trying to conform to the structure of others; she was criticized either way. In addition, she felt powerless to stand up to those authority figures who bullied her without trying to understand what she needed to thrive or valuing her efforts. Nidhi had a true warrior spirit - she fought through illness, pain, exhaustion, and disappointments, all without leaning upon anyone. Yet no one, not even Nidhi, appreciated her grit, determination, and ability to navigate her life alone. The thought, "*Why am I never good enough*?" haunted her. Metaphorically, Nidhi gulped all of that criticism down and it was all stored in her subconscious.

Our last session was deep and cathartic. We went through each memory of being criticized and judged, releasing those undigested emotions which were tainting those memories like tearing pages from an old file sitting in the subconscious library, creating space for a new, empty book to write new goals, desires, and aspirations. She also remembers the affirmation she created for herself at our last session: "*To get married.*" That was a mantra I asked her to affirm during self-hypnosis for twenty-one days, which is the time it takes to create new neuropathways in the brain. Nidhi diligently followed all the suggestions I gave her post session. To bring about new behavior and shifts it's crucial to understand the power of repetition. In post session, the person is asked to repeat the new chosen positive affirmations in the mind to create a new neural network that generates a positive energy flow, creating excitement and motivation to reach the desired goals.

It was almost miraculous how, after that last session, Nidhi started to shed weight without much effort.

Shortly after that, she met the perfect person and became engaged. It's funny - she actually saw her future husband during one of her sessions. She knew him and had dated him years before, but they had lost touch and she had no current romantic connection with him. Within a few months post session, he spontaneously reconnected with her through social media; they dated and got married.

I spoke with Nidhi recently, and she had this to say:

"You really, really changed my life. After I came back from my sister's house, I started shedding weight. It seemed like magic. My relatives could not believe it was me because I had lost so much. I got the best compliment ever when my family told me I looked like my sister- someone I had been negatively compared to my whole life! When I went on my honeymoon, I wore a miniskirt I hadn't worn since before my thyroid diagnosis, ten or twelve years back, and it fit!"

CHAPTER THREE

THE OUTCOME

I tell Nidhi's story all the time, because it both changes the way we look at weight issues and it highlights the devastating effects of judging others. I also tell it because it showcases what I have seen to be true over and over again. When we go through catharsis of negative emotions of the past, we not only clear up the problem we came to solve, we tend to shift everything else in our lives that isn't working as well. I call this *the ripple effect.*

Health, relationships, jobs and careers, goals and goal attainment - all of these things tend to transform almost overnight when this modality is used as a healing tool. Your mind has so much power. When all of that old baggage of the past is cast away then new things, new possibilities, can enter. Once your subconscious is released from negative emotions, it becomes almost effortless to get what you want.

In Nidhi's case, not only did she lose weight but the man who would be her husband could finally reconnect with her - as if he had just been waiting for her to be ready.

Her career shifted, too. Nidhi was indirectly pushed into teaching, but it was not her true passion. Once our sessions were complete and she returned to her old job, it just didn't feel right. This is what she shared:

"I interviewed for a job with an online-based education company and I got the job. After some of my colleagues got to know me, they started encouraging me to do my own writing. Last year, I started my blog. I finally understood that I had to realize my own worth, my own desires and to do my own work. I have had so many positive comments. I write with my heart about my experiences and people really get something from it. Though I no longer care what people think, some of my readers tell me my writing has changed their lives. And I love it, love it!"

I remember her sister coming back to me after Nidhi's sessions saying, "*You have transformed my sister. She is a completely different person.*" But that's not actually true. Nidhi isn't a different person; she is now her *own* person! She is true to herself without trying to contort into anyone else's version of what her life should look like. Her true self was hidden under all that anger, frustration, and criticism she got from her family and her environment. Now that true fighter, that soldier, that person who just goes for it, is in charge. As a result, she moves through her life with ease. Now when she puts in even a little effort, she gets the results she wants. Nidhi's case exemplifies what can happen when we step into our true selves and live our lives like no one is watching!

Eventually her most difficult relationships with the family members who were so critical of her changed, too. Now that Nidhi charts her own course, the criticism comes far less often, and when it does, she lets it roll off her back. It no longer destroys her confidence or changes her path.

"Hypnotherapy is a powerful tool that brings us to our unadulterated essence, free from the tapes and training of others. Once that is achieved, our body restores its unique blueprint of true health."

CHAPTER FOUR

SONIA: HOOKED ON HYPNOTHERAPY

"The body says what the mind cannot."

During my hypnotherapy training, I was asked to participate in a demonstration of a new technique. The facilitator asked me what issue I wanted to work on, and I happily said, "*I have no issues. Life is good*!" I remember everyone in class looked at me with raised eyebrows as if to say, *"Is she in denial?"* Because I felt this was an opportunity to experience something new, I chose to work on a weird, very specific anxiety I had experienced for years.

I used to feel really nervous whenever I was in a parking garage or other place at night when there was no one around. This happened often after finishing up a late evening clinic shift when the streets were empty and the parking garage was deserted. I'm not a person who gets scared easily and these were always well-lit spaces in fairly quiet neighborhoods. Yet my sense was that I was always looking behind me, as if someone else was there; and I didn't like that feeling.

So, I told my facilitator about the issue and proudly explained that I already knew the reason for it. I had figured out while sitting in class that it was connected to an incident I experienced in my childhood. She said, "*OK, you know the reason and yet you still feel this way. Would you like to work on this*?" And I realized that I very much did.

Under hypnosis, the therapist took me back to the episode that I knew was at the heart of this anxiety. It happened when I was twelve years old. Sunday night was movie night in our household. In fact, Sunday nights in Delhi were movie nights for pretty much the entire city. Families would be glued to the T.V. as networks broadcasted really nice family movies starting at 6 p.m. The roads and sidewalks would be deserted as the glare of T.V. screens could be seen in almost every open living room window.

I am the eldest child and a true foodie at heart. I was always coming up with the perfect foods for any occasion. So that particular night, I was craving my favorite street food from a place we visited often. My mom was giving me a hard time about being so picky, but I was insistent, and so she let me go on my quest.

There was no fear about going out alone. Back then I didn't think the vendor's stall was very far from the house, but now I realize that it kind of was. It was probably half a kilometer or so from home. I remember noticing just how quiet my neighborhood was during my walk. There wasn't a single soul out in the streets, but I wasn't anxious. After all that, I reached the vendor's stall and discovered that the vendor wasn't there! Of course! He was probably at home watching movies with his own family. By now, it was dark outside, and I was pretty bummed that I couldn't get my favorite snacks; but the street lights were on, and I happily skipped back to my snug home and family.

As I arrived home and began to climb the stairs to our walk up on the second floor, I sensed a male figure behind me. I didn't really think anything about it - we lived in a five-story building with many apartments, so it was no big deal to meet someone else on the stairs. But just as I got to our door and put my hand up to ring the bell, the man grabbed me from behind, putting his mouth on my face and his hand on my chest. I screamed, "*MOM*!" And when I screamed, he ran away.

Re-experiencing this childhood event within the safety of a hypnotherapy session was interesting. It seemed so real, and I was able to recall all of these individual moments, strung together, that hadn't leeched into my consciousness before. I remember my mom and dad came running. First, mom went out into the street, asking neighbors if they had seen the stranger. When she came back with no luck, they hunkered down to determine the best course of action. All that time I just kept crying.

During the exercise, I was distinctly aware of my emotions. I was so afraid, I was crying like a baby - that gasping cry that little kids do. To heal this fear, under hypnosis as guided by my facilitator, I met that younger self as the adult of today - and it was so powerful to comfort this younger, scared self! *"I am here, I am listening to you, I understand you, I know the fear was so big in you."* I also realized that because my parents were incredibly frightened themselves, they focused their actions on finding the man. They were kind, loving, and attentive; but no one spoke a word. And their unspoken concern just didn't register with my younger self, in part because she was so scared and possibly in a state of shock.

So, during this session, I got the opportunity to have this conversation with my parents (within my subconscious mind) in order to give that twelve-year-old self the chance to heal. In that moment, as I looked at my parents as an adult, I immediately understood that my parents expressed their care and concern through their actions that night. The most cathartic moment for me was knowing, without a doubt, that taking measures to make sure this stranger never accosted me again was the language of love they knew! As I explained how I felt that night when no words were spoken, I sensed as if hearing me say that made my parents cry. I could feel their helplessness. With that catharsis, something shifted within me, as though my younger self understood that entire night in a new way. The session closed with a beautiful embrace from my loving parents and my 12-year-old self feeling safe and secure once again.

I was so surprised by the instant change in me afterwards. Truthfully, I tested it out a few times. I would park my car on an empty street and think, *"Let's see what happens,"* then check in with myself. *"OK Sonia, how are you feeling? Do you want to look behind you?"* I realized after a few times doing this that I really didn't care anymore. Within a few weeks, I had actually forgotten that I used to react in that tensed-up way whenever I was in a place like that.

That random demonstration during a hypnotherapy training course was a turning point for me. It really highlighted the intensity of how experiences from our past can show up in the present. That day I said I had no issues... Oh well, I was indeed in denial! Since that training six years ago I have done nonstop work on myself in order to understand the effects of negative programs playing in my subconscious.

"I believe we are all project in making and each therapeutic dip in the subconscious brings out a better, more complete version of our own selves. And that is exactly what got me hooked on hypnotherapy!"

CHAPTER FIVE

GRACE: DESPERATE FOR SLEEP

"I don't know what will happen if I close my eyes."

THE PROBLEM

When I met Grace, she appeared as an immaculately dressed and very put-together woman. You would never know that she had been struggling with both insomnia and migraines for almost two decades. She averaged two to three hours of light sleep each night and had difficulty in both falling asleep and waking up without being able to fall back to sleep. She woke up tired, drained, and cloudy-headed most days. She also struggled with anxiety and depression- two conditions linked to chronic insomnia in the medical literature.

Grace is a woman with resources and is, to some extent, in the public eye. Given her fortunate circumstances, she is deeply committed to giving back and spends a significant amount of time doing charity work. This means she frequently gives speeches and hosts events - but her insomnia and migraines combined to make her feel anxious, restless, and jittery. She somehow managed, until she experienced a wakeup call (pun intended). Grace was driving with her husband and young son in the car and fell asleep at the wheel for a few seconds. Fortunately, no disaster happened; they just went off the road and ended up in a field. Everyone was fine, but the close call shocked her into making a fervid commitment to resolving her insomnia.

After multiple visits with her primary care physician failed to restore her sleep, she saw two sleep specialists, had her circadian rhythm checked, implemented a strict sleep schedule, and maintained meticulous sleep hygiene (eye mask, ear plugs, comfortable bedding, cool and dark room, limited caffeine and alcohol). She tried multiple prescription medications, and though they helped, she hated the thought of becoming dependent on them, so she kept looking for alternatives. She exercised in sunlight daily and tried multiple supplements, CBD and THC, essential oils, cognitive behavioral therapy, and different types of meditation.

Though Grace is a successful professional with above-average intelligence, connected to excellent medical resources, and consistent in her efforts, nothing she did succeeded in improving her sleep.

CHAPTER FIVE

THE SESSION

As she enters into hypnosis, I ask Grace to become aware of the reason for her insomnia. Within a few moments, she views herself at age four in a strange hospital room. Her mom is there, too, crying nonstop. There are all these people buzzing around and Grace is scared that she will never see her mom again. She says, "*The surgeons are coming to take me away*." Grace immediately understands that this memory stems from the heart surgery she had at that age to repair a defect she was born with.

As they wheel her into the operating room, she is terrified. Everyone she sees has masks on. "*I am looking at my mom, but no one is telling me anything. No one is even talking to me*." The last thing she hears is, "*Close your eyes,*" as a mask comes towards her own face. "*Whoa,*" she thinks, "*I don't know what will happen if I close my eyes! Will I see my mom again? Will I die?*" After the session, Grace realizes that, all of these years later, these are the thoughts she connects with every time she tries to fall asleep. "*I go to sleep and I don't know what's going to happen.*"

So, it was obvious that the task at hand was to release the fear, heal the emotional trauma of that surgery, and give that child a sense of calm. This is how it was done. I tell her, "*I want you to help that little girl as the surgeons take her away. You, the adult, are next to her. Only she can sense your presence; you are invisible to others. As they are putting her on the operating table and they are placing the mask on her, hold her hand and keep telling her, 'It's O.K. I'm right here. You are safe... Sleep.'"*

THE OUTCOME

A few days later, I received the following email:

Dr. Sonia,

Another good night's sleep! I fell asleep rather quickly and slept through the night until 5 a.m.! And, no headache this morning!

xoxo

This case hit me hard as a doctor. I would have never imagined that an event that occurred when Grace was four years old could be responsible for *decades of suffering*. As a medical professional, to sense the power of expression and words spoken and unspoken, shook me to my core. I couldn't help but wonder what would have been the outcome if Grace's medical team had spoken to the little kid to explain what was happening.

It's easy in a hospital to think that words, body language, and facial expressions are superfluous. Yet Grace's case taught me how very important it is to reassure my patients - even if it requires extra time. In fact, I feel that we should have a mandatory *"Reassurance protocol"* as guidance for medical teams to deliver to every patient who gets diagnosed with a chronic disease or is going for a surgery or a procedure. Just to say, *"Everything is going to be OK... You will be fine,"* and to mean it by making an eye contact, is like giving a hypnotic suggestion... it can perhaps prevent some other Grace from getting insomnia.

Why not say these words and mean them - even when there is a poor prognosis? We've all had our own stories, and read them in the medical literature, of miraculous healings that couldn't have occurred – yet they did. Who are we to take away hope? Even so, hope isn't necessarily about living or dying; sometimes hope is about sensing that someone has our back, even as the world is falling down around us.

At medical school I wasn't taught to be concerned about the ways my patients feel in a situation they find themselves in. I wasn't schooled to tell the truth while also letting them know I had their back. I wasn't trained to ask, *"How am I being?"* or to understand that this is almost as important as what I am doing. I wasn't trained to understand my patients' emotional needs. It didn't dawn on me that my patients could sense my energy without me saying a word.

"Grace's experience opened me up to a new knowing and reiterated the power of words and being human! It's time to integrate that missing human BEING in Medicine."

CHAPTER SIX

SONIA: SOMETHING IS MISSING

"Recognizing that disease can be impacted by a patient's emotions and past experiences - THIS is patient-centered care."

When I went to medical school, I dreamed of all the patients I could help. I studied hard so I could understand the body and its workings, identify problems, and cure those problems once I diagnosed them. But after fifteen years of practicing medicine, I noticed that many of my patients would come in with similar complaints that were generally centered around one or more of these symptoms: pain, exhaustion, gastric problems, mood swings, weight gain, sexual dysfunction, depression and anxiety. Despite treatment, they would often come in with a new complaint on top of the old one that had never resolved, and they kept asking me what else they could do. Typically, I had already exhausted my diagnostics and prescribed medications. And that look on their faces - that mixture of desperation, anger, sadness, and profound helplessness - made me start to feel like I was missing something. Sure, I could give a diagnosis of exclusion, like fibromyalgia or chronic fatigue syndrome; but those diagnoses are designed to assist with reimbursement more than the treatment and cure of the patient. Another prescription meant I was treating a symptom without ever reaching the cause.

In truth, being aware of our patient's emotional lives benefits us, as well. In med school, most of us learned to disconnect from our *own* emotions. While this ideal was presented to us as a way of staying professional, clear-headed, and calm in a crisis, I'm not sure it has served us all that well. Experiences create emotions that can have a lifelong impact - both negative and positive. Uncovering those emotions that cause negative feedback loops of suffering and unhappiness can protect doctors against burnout, help us create a better balance between personal and professional, and generally make us happier people. Hypnotherapy has brought home to me the realization that doctors need and deserve healing, too.

I began to have the distinct impression that there was a void in my knowledge which created my frustration. I also began to understand that my frustration was actually sadness and helplessness in disguise - which seemed to echo the feelings of my patients. So, I started to really look at my practice, both the way I was taught to treat patients, and their overall level of health. I also worked to consciously connect with the feeling I had every time I wrote a prescription for something chronic. I became clear about several things: that there are major limitations in medical science; that I had failed to actually care for my patients the way I had hoped to in med school; that writing prescriptions and "managing" illness gave me an incomplete sense of success as a doctor; and that I had replaced the word "*cure*" with the word "*treatment.*" In terms of chronic disease, "cure" had become a four-letter word. But I refused to accept that there was nothing I could do. So I began to search for a way to shift my practice.

I started by asking myself questions. What if the burden of not making my patients truly well is the real reason for my job dissatisfaction? What would my day look like if I didn't write a prescription for many of my patients, but instead enabled them to walk out of my office without their symptoms and nothing in their hands except their bag or coat? Better yet, what would that *feel* like? I found that the solution to both my own burnout, and that of my patients, was so brilliantly simple.

Let's say, in an emergency room rotation one evening, a car accident victim comes in with a bleeding injury. How will it be if only replacement fluids are transfused to manage this patient, and suturing the wound is completely omitted? It seems ridiculous in the face of a critical care example - yet we do this very same thing with our chronically ill patients. *We only treat the symptoms and fail to ameliorate the cause.*

Most doctors would agree that writing a prescription isn't the reason that got them into medicine. We dreamed of having a real relationship with our patients, making the correct diagnosis *through that relationship*, and offering a way back to good health. Sure, chronic illness is complicated. Stress, mental illness, the physical and emotional demands of work and family life, spiritual angst, lack of exercise, genetics, and diet all play a part of both contracting an illness and successfully overcoming it. These factors are multidimensional – encompassing the biological, psychosocial, and spiritual elements of a patient's life - yet we do not take a multidimensional approach to treatment. We live in an assembly-line system of care that (more often than we care to admit) addresses the physiological causes of disease without taking into account the psychosocial stressors, thoughts, and emotions of our patients. Yes, we might suggest they check out a therapist, gym, or yoga studio; but from my vantage point, this doesn't appear to empower doctors or patients.

This may be a revolutionary viewpoint, but when we fail to alleviate the pain and suffering of our patients - despite the very latest advances in medical sciences - we add to our own stress as physicians. Many of us share a feeling that there are things in modern medicine that have to change. Yet, given the fact that it takes decades for new research to catch up to the way we practice, we could be waiting a pretty long time.

Fortunately, there are new sciences - quantum physics, epigenetics and metagenomics - that are pushing us to ask some important new questions. *"Can I envision a different kind of healthcare? What are we missing? What am I yearning for as a physician, as a patient? If I had it, how would it make me feel? Would it feel empowering? Can we view results of any new modality as viable, based on the results?"*

As someone who is on the other side of these questions, I see all of us as frogs in a well. We see what we see, and it's fine; but when we use our innate strength to jump out of that well, we glimpse a brighter, more beautiful, more expansive world. If we want to reshape modern medicine into a system that treats chronic illness as successfully as it does acute medical conditions, we must take a more holistic approach. Acknowledging the mind/body connection, and adding tools that address it, is a good start. This is the beginning of true patient-centered care.

My life today, the way I think about healing, and the way I choose to help people, have all drastically changed. I finished my first hypnotherapy training six years ago; and since then, I haven't stopped moving forward with this incredible therapy. I've helped hundreds of patients heal from chronic diseases, pain, and mental distress that hadn't responded to traditional medical treatment.

This is now my passion and my mission.

*"Finally, I am curing;
finally, I am healing. I am treating
the cause and not just the symptom.
The void is filled!"*

FREE RESOURCE

Watch this video on "The Power of Words" to better understand hypersuggesstibility for physicians and healthcare professionals.

https://www.enso-nia.com/within/resources

CHAPTER SEVEN

SUSANNE: THE SAVIOR WITHIN

"I have difficulty digesting life."

THE PROBLEM

Susanne is an eloquent, graceful, and beautiful woman in her late forties, she has delicate features and appears very feminine. She books a session with me because she has longstanding gut issues that have created all kinds of problems in her life. Her original diagnoses are chronic gastritis and esophagitis; but later on she is also diagnosed with Irritable Bowel Syndrome (IBS) and H. pylori - a type of bacteria that can infect the digestive tract, creating various symptoms and increasing a patient's risk of getting stomach cancer.

Due to the H. pylori, her doctors have deemed her a cancer risk; so she is receiving a multi-course antibiotic treatment with follow-ups every six months, as well as an annual endoscopy. When I meet

Susanne, she has been treating the H. pylori for over a year. Though she has been very proactive about her own health, has made significant lifestyle changes (including a very strict diet, supplementation, and sleep hygiene), and has seen numerous specialists, these efforts have not yielded results.

In our intake, she tells me a bit about her life. By now, her stomach issues are so severe that she inevitably has to run to the restroom with diarrhea during any meeting or presentation at work. She agonizes every single night about how she will get through the next day. This nightly worry routine eventually leads to *insomnia*. She also talks about *anxiety and panic attacks*, which she connects not only to the IBS but to a long-standing feeling of being judged. The *anxiety* worsens after she is assigned to a new department within her company. *Depression* arrives when she has to curtail her friendships and social outings because it becomes so hard to cope with her IBS in public. This is devastating; Suzanne is a highly social person with lots of friends and enjoys nights out and new experiences.

She has tried everything regarding her gut. She has gone gluten-free, eats a vegan diet, has regular endoscopies, is on a year-long antibiotic course for the H. pylori, and exercises regularly - yet she feels no better. Though she looks younger than her stated age, she feels much older and shares that her life is completely dominated by her stomach.

In talking about her childhood, Susanne divulges that she was an unplanned and unwanted pregnancy. Her mother attempted to hide the pregnancy with the notion of giving her up for adoption, but her grandparents found out and stepped in to raise her. For the first four years, she was in a pretty loving situation. She saw her mom frequently, but her grandparents were her essential caregivers. That all changed when Susanne's mom got re-married; then, Suzanne went to live with her mom and new stepfather.

She also recalls that her relationship with her mom has always been strained, in large part because her mom is really controlling. This has always been the case, but it worsened when Susanne became a teenager. "*There is no flexibility, no choice is ever given to me. She always makes the choice for me.*" She is treated like a child to the point that, when the grandmother that helped raise her dies while Susanne is away at college, her mom doesn't even tell her - because she "didn't want to disturb her studies." Suzanne is shattered by not getting to say good-bye or to be with her beloved grandmother as she passes. This is one example in a long line of choices that her mom makes for her.

In this pre-session meeting, she says two interesting things that act as clues to her underlying issues. The first is this statement: "*I feel I have difficulty digesting life.*" Fascinating, given her host of stomach issues. Secondly, the words, "*unwanted and unloved,*" come up more than once. These two breadcrumbs along the path of her psyche tell me exactly how we need to start our sessions.

THE SESSIONS

During our first two sessions, under hypnosis, Susanne is able to communicate with all the people in her life who have caused her to feel unwanted and unloved, as well as review the situations that have created an inability to digest life (literally). As I guide her into her subconscious, she dialogues with all of these people (her mom, an aunt, some girlfriends from high school, an ex-boyfriend, and a close friend). Because she is in a safe space in her own mind, she can now tell them all of the things she didn't have the courage or words for at the time. These powerful interactions include the adult Susanne telling her mom with force: "*I deserve to exist!*" She also has a heartbreaking conversation with the grandmother she wasn't ready to lose. "*I am running into her arms. She is telling me she is proud of the choices I have made, that I am enough. She reminds me that she has never really left. She tells me, 'I am always here.'*" After these interactions, she can literally sense what she calls "*toxic energies*" moving out of her body. "*They're moving out of my head, my heart, my stomach and my gut. They represent self-doubt, unworthiness, not being loved, not being accepted, not being enough.*"

I also ask Susanne to sense that part of herself that feels unwanted and unloved. "*Imagine that part of yourself in front of you.*" I am surprised to hear her say, "*I am one year old.*" In order to make this little one feel safe, I ask the adult Susanne to tell this very young child,

"I want you and I finally found you. I am here to give you that unconditional love you so deserve." As Susanne talks to her younger self, this moment is touching and cathartic; the child is able to connect with an unconditional love that she now knows is always with her. A new foundation of "self-love" was laid there.

After we complete these two complex sessions, more clarity and awareness start to flow. She senses that things are already different. She tells me, *"There is an awareness that things are shifting already. I feel I can flow. I want to digest life with ease; I want to feed on love."* This phrase, *"I want to digest life with ease; I want to feed on love"* becomes her mantra for the next twenty-one days.

As Susanne enters hypnosis in our third meeting, I begin by asking her to sense that young child who feels not good enough. Susanne finds herself as a schoolgirl, age five or six, who feels she doesn't belong. Her mom and her mom's husband are talking about whether he will adopt Susanne, and whether or not they should have a baby together. During her intake, Susanne tells me that she did become a big sister at the age of ten. At first she was so excited – but she quickly began to feel that her mom, stepdad, and sister are the "real" family and she is just an interloper. *"I don't belong."* As we navigate this in our session, I ask Susanne, *"You want to be a part of this family, but you feel like you don't belong. So, what are you deciding?"* Her quiet response is, *"I will try to be a good girl. I will keep giving so hopefully one day, I will be seen, and I will receive."*

Susanne's need to give to everyone around her – along with a deep-seated sense of being unworthy to receive - became obvious. Susanne understood this vicious circle: The more she fears she won't be loved and seen, the more she over-gives to friends and family. Then, her own sense of unworthiness stops her from receiving in return; this makes her feel not good enough, which once again makes her give more to others to seek validation. This realization was another hugely cathartic moment for her. For the first time, she fully understood her behavior.

"It was so clear to Susanne that this child represented her inner strength that had gotten locked in time and space. Finally, she had unlocked that part."

This moment is nothing less than transformative. After this session, Susanne reports that, right away, she has a lot of relief from her digestive issues. *"It seems like a dark, swirling energy has left my gut. All those times that others have made me feel self-doubt, unworthiness, all of those times I had to do more in order to be acknowledged - it's like those murky vapors are moving out. I now sense inner stability and strength."* In an email she sends me within a few days of this session, she writes, *"I feel fantastic! There are times now that I don't even think of my stomach. This is so unusual."*

In our final and most fascinating session, we work within the hypnotic state to clear the cellular memory of these negative emotions from the digestive tract – a technique known as *organ regeneration*, where the power of mind is used to reset the body to its functional and original blueprint. To begin, I ask Susanne to see, in her mind's eye, her entire digestive system in front of her and to let me know how it looks. She does this easily.

So, I continue to guide her, "Imagine that you are a skilled surgeon, and you are doing surgery on your digestive tract to remove what you feel doesn't seem right. To remove it, you will use your imagination." And Susanne did exactly that, cleaning up the image of the diseased organs through creative imagination under hypnosis.

As Susanne moves into her stomach, she says, "I see two things that look like small tumors with high acidity and erosions." At this point, she begins to cry saying, "This is so creepy because I see eyes. Little things that are sticking to the membranes that look like eyes. They are crawling and holding onto my stomach with claws. They are even between the linings of my stomach. They are sneaky and trying to hide."

This description of eyes in her stomach sounds like a very good layperson's description of highly resistant H. pylori bacteria as seen in a gram stain under a microscope.

Susanne continues her healing journey by focusing on the two tumors, which she removes with a scalpel. She then uses a sandblaster on the "*eyes*" saying, "*There are so many of them. They are all over my stomach. I just keep cleaning and cleaning.*"

It takes her awhile and when she is done with this, I instruct Susanne to sense the template of a healthy stomach coming to her, describing it as "*a new cover, a new healthy blueprint, that you give to your stomach.*" I ask her how it looks and feels. "*The sensations are so real - it feels like a beautiful cooling sensation. It's as if I am getting a completely new digestive tract. There is new joy and a love of being in this body which comes from acceptance and an inner peace and calm.*"

THE OUTCOME

Shortly after this last session, Susanne not only feels fantastic, but she radically changes her life. She realizes that she is in a toxic work environment and decides to quit her job. Surprisingly, she then moves back to her home country and lives with her mom for a while. This turns out to be a really good thing. "*We have a completely different relationship now.*"

But the best news - her next follow up endoscopy, which is done sometime just after our last session, shows a miraculous improvement. All of the erosions and the H. pylori are gone! Her gastroscopy report shows a normal and healthy digestive tract. "*Pylori eradication is confirmed.*" The recommendation from her physician is for a follow up endoscopy in one to two years.

Though her medical issues were certainly complex, she is markedly better after six hypnotherapy sessions held within a three-month period.

Here is an email Susanne sent me six months after our last session...

Hi Sonia,

Reading your email made me reflect upon where I was one year ago, when I was processing emotions of my inner child and teenage self. I have such a strong vision of the energetic surgery we did on my physical body, and 'sand blasting' those thousands of 'eyes' from my stomach wall. It all seems from another life.

I've come to celebrate the death of who I was, and embrace how I've become closer to my true self, having made some dramatic changes."

Thank you for being my navigator through those times when I faced true panic and distress. I no longer take prescription sleeping pills. I rely on melatonin, exercise, outdoors, and eating well to improve my sleep, along with a simple daily life. I feel great and I can eat anything I want without stomach issues.

Susanne

I was so in awe of Susanne, the way she could see her disease through her mind's eye. She had no medical knowledge and had done no research on anatomy or H. pylori, yet her representations were incredibly accurate. Her mind just showed her the right pictures. She was able to see the bacteria clinging with all its might to her mucosa, as well as the lesions, nodules, and pus-like sludge within the digestive tract. She could imagine using tools similar to those used by surgeons to remove what she saw, quickly and efficiently.

When I met Susanne, she felt helpless in the wake of her own suffering. She had done so much and yet her health had only worsened. But with the help of her subconscious, she became her own liberator. After working with hundreds of patients using hypnotherapy, I have no doubt that we can all achieve this mastery.

> "OUR MINDS CAN BOTH CREATE 'DIS-EASE' AND HEAL IT."

CHAPTER EIGHT

HYPNOTHERAPY: IT BELONGED TO US

"The aware physician
must be alert to any development
that will increase his understanding.
When a new method or treatment
consistently gets impressive results, it
is the responsibility of every
doctor to take notice."

~ Morris Netherton

Trance – or, a state of hypnosis - is something we have all commonly experienced. If you have ever driven your car to a destination and realized you didn't remember how you got there; or you are so engrossed reading a book that you don't hear your phone ring; or you walk past a bakery and the delicious smell takes you back in in time to your grandma's kitchen when you were a child... Then you have actually experienced a light trance. Hypnosis is really nothing more than a common state of altered awareness - and some of the oldest cultures in the world have used altered states as a way to enhance life and health.

Hypnosis used to belong to the world of medicine; it used to belong to doctors. In the purview of physicians, it was used as a medical treatment for physiological and mental illness and as a highly effective anesthetic. It has survived the test of time because highly respected pioneers such as Hippocrates, Paracelsus, James Braid, Sigmund Freud, Jean-Martin Charcot, and Franz Anton Mesmer achieved, and shared, their amazing results.

Hippocrates, the physician who authored the core tenet of our doctor's oath, commonly employed what he called "trance healing" in his practice. Chiron, a Greek physician, used hypnosis as an anesthetic to perform painless surgeries. This was later replicated by the work of two Scottish physicians: John Elliotson (1791 - 1859), who in 1849 founded the first "mesmeric hospital," and James Esdaile (1808-1859). Both of these surgeons also performed countless successful operations on patients that featured hypnosis as the primary anesthetic. In the case of Esdaile, his cases even included limb amputation. Based in part on their work, the British Medical Association in 1955 officially approved hypnosis as an anesthetic for pain relief in both childbirth and surgery.

One of hypnosis' most famous practitioners, Austrian physician Franz Anton Mesmer (1734 - 1815), would hypnotize large groups of people in mass ritual ceremonies that produced many accounts of recorded healings. His use of trance stemmed from that of ancient shamans and Native American healers who successfully used a combination of chant, ceremony, and plant medicine to produce a trance-like state that led to healing. His work became so well known that we still use the word "mesmerized" today to refer to someone who appears to be in a daze, which is nothing more than a slightly altered state of consciousness (similar to what everyone does when they daydream or mentally "zone out" for a few minutes).

Because Mesmer did much of his work in France, he directly impacted the work of Jean Martin Charcot (1825 - 1893), the founder of modern neurology. Charcot reverse-engineered hypnosis to actually *produce* symptoms in his volunteers such as blindness, deafness, and paralysis, which disappeared once he brought them out of trance. He was a very visible teacher who gave many lectures and demonstrations to students and physicians.

Dr. James Braid (1795 - 1806), considered the father of modern hypnosis, was the one who actually coined the term "hypnosis" based on the Greek god of sleep, Hypnos. Though he was initially exposed to hypnosis through the vaudevillian-type entertainers who used it as a stage act, he recognized that it could be put to a medicinal use. Through his extensive experimentation and studies, he treated a wide variety of conditions, including a 45-year-old man who suffered a spinal cord injury that caused pain and limited mobility in his upper body. Braid so successfully used hypnosis to treat the condition that the man went back to work after two months of daily sessions. His patients also included stroke victims and patients with paralysis and headaches.

Dr. Braid's most important contribution was the discovery that contradicted the idea that people in trance were "asleep." He recognized that people in trance were actually very aware, noting that *"hearing in the trance state is about twelve times more acute than everyday consciousness*." He also observed that autonomic processes like heart rate and blood circulation could be controlled during hypnosis. Because of these findings, it was his strong belief that hypnosis should only be used by medical professionals. His research, along with the groundbreaking, prolific, and timeless research of Milton Erickson, provided the foundation of what we consider the modern uses of hypnotism in medical and psychological treatment.

Milton Erickson was a well-known American psychiatrist, psychologist, and founder of the American Society for Clinical Hypnosis. At age 17, he contracted polio and was severely paralyzed. Doctors believed he would die. While recovering in bed, unable to move or speak, he became strongly aware of the significance of nonverbal communication, including body language and tone of voice. He also began to have "body memories" of the muscular activity of his own body; by concentrating on those memories he slowly regained control and movement of the paralyzed parts. Eventually, he was able to talk, use his arms, and walk with a cane. Over a 50-year career span he conducted extensive research on suggestion and hypnosis. The Ericksonian approach departs from traditional hypnosis in a variety of ways. It stresses the importance of an interactive therapeutic relationship, as well as the purposeful engagement of the inner resources and experiential life of the patient. This revolutionized the practice of hypnotherapy.

So why did hypnosis cease to be a part of our practice? Does it have to do with the vaudevillian entertainers (you'll remember the stories about them getting their volunteers to "cluck like a chicken") who unintentionally created fear and skepticism of hypnosis in the name of entertainment? These stage acts made it seem as if the person in trance was completely at the mercy of the hypnotic suggestion and the hypnotist. These fears became so prevalent that *hypnophobia*, or the fear of being hypnotized, was created. Combined with other political and economic factors at work, the belief that hypnosis was mysterious and scary led to a decrease in its use.

Unlike the stage hypnosis, hypnotherapy's focus is not to entertain, but to elicit healing; and (unlike the former) there is no mind control. Like physicians, hypnotherapists work within a set of ethics that includes the bedrock of our physician's oath: "Do no harm."

There are some who believe that hypnosis "plants" false memories. However, the essence of the altered state itself means that patients are aware of everything that is happening. Our ethics compel us, in every session, to empower the patient to find their own solution;

to take only those actions that feel comfortable to them; and to envision the future that they want to see for themselves. The hypnotherapist is always working within the confines of a patient's own free will. Yes, a hypnotherapist sometimes has to facilitate re-scripting of bad memories to bring about a shift - but it's this new perspective, achieved in trance, that provides innumerable benefits to the patient. It is the patients themselves who create these new scenarios. Hypnotherapists assist their patients with uncovering unhealthy themes and patterns, empower them to overcome those themes and patterns, and guide them in digesting negative emotion. This is no different than the goals of cognitive therapy.

The genius of hypnosis is its ability to bypass the defense mechanisms of the conscious mind in order to work directly with the subconscious. Bad habits, phobias, blocks, pain, illness, and self-sabotage can all be signs that there are archived aspects of ourselves that need to be healed. When we tap into the subconscious, they are readily available and amenable to change.

Thankfully, hypnosis survived the test of time and today it is once again beginning to get recognition as a legitimate treatment in medicine, psychology, and dentistry. Many highly acclaimed research and educational institutions now offer seminars and training courses in hypnotherapy. Numerous studies are exploring the use of hypnotherapy in some surprising ways. Hypnotherapy is, after all, a patient-centered treatment that takes into account a patient's unique set of life circumstances, the power of their own mind, and their own fervent wishes and desires.

"As physicians we desperately need a bridge between the medicine of the past and the medicine of the future."

I am convinced that hypnotherapy is that bridge. It is a simple, elegant solution that is effective and easy to integrate. It gives physicians the ability to be creative, to heal when we couldn't before, and to connect with our patients in a way that we haven't in a long time.

"Hypnotherapy can affect miraculous change within the physiology without the use of anything but words, images, and relaxation – and without side effects or the need for a lifetime of treatment. It's time that we doctors remember our history."

"IT'S TIME TO RECLAIM WHAT HAS ALWAYS BEEN OURS!"

CHAPTER NINE

SONIA: THE PHYSICIAN SHIFTS

"When the Physician felt stuck, the Hypnotherapist said: Bring it on!"

When I stumbled into hypnotherapy, it most certainly didn't disappoint. I jumped into training and was so excited that, even before I finished, I was already wondering how to broach the subject of bringing it into my work with my medical patients. Serendipitously, a local radio show made this much easier.

I was in training for the last level of my certification program when I got a call from the show's host, who used to have me on as a guest speaker pretty frequently. The show was typical - I would man the microphone as the public called in to ask me their medical questions. Rob, the radio host, called me to say that he had an unexpected opening on his show the next day, and wondered if I could take the hour-long slot. Fortunately, my trainer flexed the next day's curriculum so I could appear on the program.

Mind you, I had no thought of talking about hypnotherapy at all - I was just going to do my normal thing as a physician, answering questions about trending illnesses, new medications, and whatever else came up. But when I called Rob back to let him know I would be on the segment, I happened to mention that I was doing this amazing course. Now, Rob loves to riff, and I love that energy as well; so he feels pretty comfortable asking me random questions on air. Even so, I wasn't even remotely prepared for him to ask me, on live radio, about my training!

"*So Doc,*" he says, "*You are learning hypnotherapy?*" And I say laughing, "*I haven't even told my own colleagues I 'm learning this and you ask me on live radio!*" But I got on a roll, talking about the mind and what kind of results hypnotherapy produces. The phone lines started to light up. People were calling to ask all kinds of questions, including: "*Where is this doctor who is practicing this?*" I'm telling you, the whole segment was on fire! We got so many calls that when I came out of the booth, the producer told me he wanted to put me on a two-hour segment in an even more popular time slot in the coming weeks with the same topic.

I still didn't know how I was going to integrate this into my practice at the time; but because of that radio segment, within three days I had my first patient. After hearing me on the radio, parents of a teenaged boy called me to explain that the bullying their son had experienced at school resulted in depression and anxiety that had so far been unchanging to treatment. He had tried medications, but none of them were working. My heart went out to them. They felt so strongly that I could help, and they were sitting in front of me with those imploring eyes. I just couldn't say no. Fortunately, the head of my medical practice was an open-minded leader. I told him about the radio show and the parents who had approached me about their son. At the time, I was working under a contract with a fixed salary and hours, so the solution was pretty straightforward. My medical director created a new contract so that I could deliver so many hours as a physician and so many hours as a hypnotherapist. It also allowed me to use the clinic's facilities.

At the time, I couldn't believe it was that easy. I wanted to practice both, and I got both! I became the first doctor in Dubai to combine mainstream medical practice with hypnotherapy services at the same clinic. I know now that when you are at the right place at the right time, the universe makes it happen. Amazingly, I was given a dedicated room just for hypnotherapy, with a special couch for my patients; and I basically got free rein to discuss this treatment option with my patients as I felt appropriate. If I believed that hypnotherapy was a viable alternative, I could offer them the choice of either standard medical treatment or hypnotherapy. And slowly but surely, my hypnotherapy clients increased. I had such trust in my patients, and they in me, that when I suggested it might be time to shift to the couch, they would simply say, "*OK.*"

After combining traditional medicine and hypnotherapy for several months, even my colleagues started referring patients to me because I continued to get such positive results with atypical patients.

As I was accumulating results and confidence in my hypnotherapy practice, I began to easily enter the exam room with both modalities in mind, taking in the information my patients provided, digesting it, and then reconnecting it in a way that would allow me to combine the best of both to achieve healing. What I didn't realize at first was that the physician in me was shifting.

I vividly remember seeing a young female who came into the clinic for chest pain. Looking at her medical records I noticed that she had visited the practice four times in less than two weeks with the same complaint; and every time the ECG was done, along with other diagnostic tests to rule out cardiac versus gastric issues. As a protocol, during this visit the tests were repeated again and were inconclusive.

So, when I entered the examining room the physician in me was holding hands with the hypnotherapist. The first question I asked was, "How's life? Are you going through something difficult?" She burst out crying, as she was not expecting this question - no other doctor had asked her that. She then confided in me that her beloved father passed away three weeks back. She had to travel to India but was called back at work within a week. It was so clear to me that the pain she was experiencing was the pain of loss! I suggested to her that we shift to the hypnotherapy couch to understand this literal "heartache" as the medical tests were inconclusive.

Post-session, she left my room that day with a beautiful smile on her face, almost not remembering what had brought her to the clinic in the first place.

"And that's how the physician started holding hands with the hypnotherapist within, one patient at a time!"

CHAPTER TEN

GISELLE: AT FIRST BLUSH

"We don't know our own power."

THE PROBLEM

Giselle is a young professional woman in her twenties with porcelain skin and a quiet, thoughtful demeanor. She came to me with the complaint of anxiety, accompanied by profuse blushing, for the last eight years - medically diagnosed as rosacea. It had begun to seriously affect her work and she was desperate for relief.

She told me that this constant feedback loop of feeling anxious and leading to blushing began at work while she gave presentations, specifically when her bosses were in the audience. It got much worse when she was promoted to a high-ranking position about a year and a half before I met her. The blushing had become so severe that people would ask her repeatedly if she was all right. As a new and fast-rising executive at her firm, Giselle was really good at what she did, but her bosses started to question her abilities because of these physical symptoms – and that increased her stress even more. Ultimately, she began to bring her work problems home with her. She admitted to getting angry at her husband for small things that wouldn't normally bother her, so it had now affected her marriage, too. Her self-esteem was beginning to take a real hit.

During our intake session, she told me she grew up in an Islamic country with highly rigid societal norms. Her parents, constantly concerned about outward appearances, were extremely critical of their children. Her dad was that silent judge - he would give "the look" that would put her instantly in her place - while her mom was inappropriately loud and physically abusive at times. Giselle, through her parents' nagging criticism, was always sensing this unseen pressure and fear of failure as she was constantly reminded of being judged by others. That feeling seemed deeply embedded in her subconscious.

THE SESSIONS

In her first session, I ask Giselle to sense that part of her who feels anxious in front of others. "*Just sense how she looks.*" I am pretty amazed when she sees herself as two or three years old, saying "*I have my thumb in my mouth. I look very scared and sad.*" I ask her to sense the presence of those people this child is so scared of. Not surprisingly, her father and mother appear.

As I encourage Giselle to express everything she has never expressed to her parents, I am expecting a lot of anger. Instead, it's fear and disappointment that comes up, particularly regarding her dad. She tells me, *"I feel as if all this energy is toxic and it is affecting me badly."* In the presence of the adult self, the child feels safe; tapping on the emotions of this younger self, Giselle expresses feelings with both parents that she had never verbalized face to face. She sensed that these toxic emotions have moved out of her body through that expression alone, and she says with wonder, *"I sense my confidence returning. I am peaceful. I actually feel as though the child who was feeling fearful now wants to go close to mom and hug her."*

As she is hugging her mom, she feels this enormous regret in her dad for his actions, so the child hugs him, too. In reality, Giselle does not remember ever getting a physical embrace from either of her parents, so this moment in trance was very special. For the first time ever, this family is relaxed and loving with each other, embracing in a group hug that anchors in a whole new relationship.

In her feedback supplied a few days later she said, "I used to freak out when I got a new assignment at work, but now it is much better. My nervousness during presentations is 70% less. Because my anxiety is so much better, the rosacea is better, too - it's much less obvious."

Since Giselle reports only a 70% improvement in her symptoms, we follow up with a second session a few weeks later. We continue to focus on her anxiety, conducting a life review in order to determine the roots of this emotion. She visits many memories, travelling back in time in which she felt fearful and uncertain in the midst of those authority figures, mainly her parents, who don't always see her or her needs. These are the scenes she recollects:

Scene 1: Terrified

Giselle sees herself as a two-year-old being held by her nanny as she witnesses a screaming match between her paternal grandfather and her mother, something that is making her extremely anxious. She is terrified someone might get hurt.

Scene 2: Powerless

Giselle is seven years old, sitting in the car with her father. As they drive down the road, they pass her maternal aunt. She remembers hiding from her aunt as they drive by because she is positive that if her father and aunt see each other, they will fight. While Dad does see her aunt, he fortunately doesn't stop the car. He does tell Giselle, however, that he doesn't want her spending time with her aunt, whom Giselle adores. At this news, she feels incredibly sad and powerless.

Scene 3: Abandoned

Giselle's subconscious takes her to a parking lot where she is sitting in the back seat of a car. In the front seat, her mom is telling her dad that she is getting remarried. Giselle says, "*I am very stressed. I don't know where I will be. I feel like I will be abandoned.*"

Scene 4: Ashamed

Giselle is eleven. Her father is screaming at her because he feels she is dressed inappropriately. "*I am wearing something that has sexy written on it.*"

Scene 5: Anxious

Giselle is at a tennis club. On the first floor there is an international tennis tournament going on, and one of her favorite players is in the competition. "*I can see him from the balcony. Everyone is giving him balls and hats to sign so I throw my hat, but it gets stuck in the balcony. I try to get it out, but I can't. I am so anxious, partly because I know my mom will beat the hell out of me if I don't have my hat; and partly because I know I will be judged by all of these people, because when my mom gets hold of me, they will think I have done something wrong.*"

Scene 6: Slapped

Giselle is at her grandparent's house and her mom is very upset. Her mother is shouting at her, and then hits her. Why? Because Giselle introduced her *step*brother to someone - and her mom didn't want anyone to *know* she was married before. *"Do you know what people will think about me?"*

Scene 7: Pressure

Giselle is seventeen. She had wanted to live in Paris since she was a young girl. She found a bachelor's program there and was accepted. Though her parents were against her going, she went anyway. Miraculously, she was able to convince her mom to financially support her. In Paris, on her first day of prep classes in her new college program, Giselle says, *"I feel the pressure of the program. Before, I didn't know what I would be facing; but now I am here, and I am sensing that this is much more than I expected. I don't want to fail. I cannot go back home. So, this is where I need to fight because no matter what, I can't fail. I am extremely anxious."*

Scene 8: Insecure

Giselle is now age nineteen and in her second year of school in Paris. She is on campus when she receives a call from her mom. *"She tells me that she will no longer support me financially. Her words are very harsh. I feel rejected, but at the same time, I want to prove to her than I can do it. I am so anxious because my future is unknown. I feel very insecure."* Once again, stress and anxiety caused by her family shakes her foundation. Yet she finds a way out; waitressing allows her to provide for herself and obtain her degree.

Later in the session, she talks about the fact that asking her parents to support her Paris studies is the first thing she has ever done for herself. She really feels the pressure of this decision, exacerbated by the lack of support, since neither parent approves of her going. She is in a new city, in a new program, on her own. She recalls feeling like it would be the end of the world to fail; like it was inevitable that she *would* fail. Her anxiety and stress were enormous. It is this Can't Fail/Will Fail energy that she brings to all of her school assignments as a student - and later on, to her work assignments as an executive.

THE OUTCOME

Giselle had two sessions with me over two months. Through the reliving of these scenes, breath work, and other processes, we were able to release all of these undigested emotions. Her feedback after these sessions was remarkable. She told me that her rosacea is so much lighter. "*It now looks as natural as blush. I proudly wear it.*" She has so much more confidence now that she is getting positive feedback from her bosses at work. Her creativity had also increased, and she had designed some very well-received campaigns. In addition, her improved work situation also meant that her marriage had improved. *"I can now be myself at home."* Giselle has never needed another session.

As a doctor, it never occurred to me that someone's parenting, cultural and religious background, socioeconomic status, or education could lead to a physical manifestation through internalized beliefs developed as a child. Yet in Giselle, this process was evident. Her learned fear of failure created a level of anxiety that triggered a physical response.

On some level, she was aware of this, too. In fact, Giselle was very clear in our intake that her anxiety and fear of failure started well before the rosacea. Yet, as a physician, I would never have thought to ask her where these emotions stemmed from. In fact, her diagnosis of rosacea actually obscured the fact that her blushing (a more accurate term) had an emotional basis alongside a physical one. Giselle's case reminds me that chronic disease doesn't usually occur as the result of one huge, momentous event. Instead, like water carving mountains, many moments in time compound to wear away the body's defenses.

The critical mind develops primarily between the ages of two and eight; but surprisingly, we don't learn discernment by doing what we are told. We learn by *observing and associating*. We watch others, we form judgements, and - here's the rub - we attach emotions to those judgments. This early process results in a well-defined filter through which all future experiences pass.

Through hypnotherapy, it was easy to see Giselle's particular filter. When she talked about her anxiety at work, she used the words, "*What will people think about me*?" - particularly as it related to her blushing. These are the same words her mother used frequently. So, Giselle wasn't giving those presentations as a grounded adult; rather, her software shifted to that of the fearful child! Particularly when presenting in front of her bosses, that anxiety and fear of authority she felt as a child automatically bubbled up, hijacking the skilled, able adult.

One of the biggest "Aha!" moments for me as a hypnotherapist was that though Giselle was clearly a strong woman - strong enough to get herself through a difficult childhood and a challenging young adulthood - she couldn't see that strength in herself. All she saw was weakness and potential failure. She looked like an adult operating in a grown-up world, yet she still felt she couldn't speak up for herself because that old tape of the child being dominated by her parents was still playing in her mind.

This is true for many of us. We can survive tremendous odds yet think that it was luck, rather than our own strengths and resources, that got us through. It is particularly difficult to have that love for, and faith in, ourselves if we didn't have parents or other important adults who instilled their love and faith in us. We see everything that happens, even the good, as a product of external circumstances. As a result, what pushes us to excel is not our own confidence, but a deep-seated fear of failure and a feeling of not being good enough. That in turn leads us to believe we must work really, really hard in order to merit our success and only others can give us approval and validation.

"This is why not feeling 'good enough' can make successful people feel like imposters."

CHAPTER ELEVEN

TAMARA: INTRACTABLE

"I sat with my anger long enough, until she told me her real name was grief."

THE PROBLEM

I meet Tamara, a successful professional, after a family member gifted her with four hypnotherapy sessions. She is middle-aged with a strong physical presence and a sharp intellect that is obvious the moment she speaks. Though she looks intense and serious, she actually has an infectious humor that is fun and light.

She comes to me with long-standing medical diagnoses that include gastritis, GERD, clinical obesity, anxiety, and depression. When we first talk, the gastritis is so bad that she can't eat most foods without problems. *"I can't eat anything without some kind of stomach upset. I swear I own stock in Rolaids."* Though she is in a good amount of physical distress, the reason she has sought me out is emotional - she complains of uncontrolled anger and bursts of rage that impact her job, her marriage, and her social life: "*I become the Incredible Hulk.*" The trigger for these bursts of anger could be almost anything - someone pulling in front of her on the freeway or a slow checkout line at the grocery store. She talks about this anger taking over more and more of her life.

During her intake, it becomes obvious to me that Tamara is in fight or flight mode all the time - and has been for forty years. Her cortisol flows like the Nile, creating a cascade of physiology that over time has created health issues - primarily from her gut, but are also likely connected to her obesity and emotional eating. Over the years she has tried meditation, medication, and naturopathic medicine; but each have failed her in their own way. As she puts it, "*It's pretty hard to meditate when you are pissed off. I need my brain [to function at work] so anti-anxiety meds didn't work for me. I understood that I ate potato chips when irritated and ice cream when depressed, but that didn't enable me to stop the behaviors. I would rather eat a good steak than sip nasty-tasting tea and take supplements as my naturopath advised.*"

THE SESSIONS

In our first session, once Tamara sinks into trance, I ask her to imagine that this part of her who feels the volcanic anger is in front of her. "*You are looking at it face to face. Just sense, how does this part look or appear to you?*" After a moment, she sees herself at her current age. "*There is a sense of rigidity about her and I feel as if something is boiling inside of her that can't be extinguished."* I am fascinated by this boiling sensation she mentions, which accurately describes how GERD and gastritis would feel. I now understand that much of Tamara's anger is unconsciously held in the gut and that her anger and stomach issues are inextricably linked. Through breathwork and suggestions we were able to extinguish that so-called boiling sensation within. Tamara felt extremely light after the session, and it was not surprising to me when she reported that her stomach was feeling the same lightness.

In our first three appointments, we also uncover the genesis of her anger. Tamara's subconscious mind traces it back to several long-ago situations that created a chain of emotions: First, a feeling that things are beyond her control; then, a sense of helplessness; and finally, frustration that over time builds to her volcanic anger.

As Tamara enters trance to understand and heal this helplessness (that is clearly linked to that anger), she sees herself at the age of five or six. She had mentioned to me earlier that she has always been fascinated by horses; in trance, she saw herself as this little kid in a pasture where there are horses. *"I love horses. There is one horse that is just galloping around, and I know he needs to be settled down, so I grab the reins to stop him. I know exactly what to do, but there is a man there who just starts yelling at me to let go."* It's notable that while she is recalling this event, her cheeks are flushed, showing a physiological response to the emotions being generated as she relives her past. It dawns on Tamara that while this man was perhaps concerned about her getting hurt, her inner child knew deep down how to handle the horse and felt extremely angry that she had to bow down to the authority of this man. Her conclusion as a child in that moment was, "No one understands me!" In fact, this is how Tamara has felt her entire life; and as her mind was showing her the memories, the realization of that childhood conclusion was dawning on the adult of now.

I then ask her to go to the next memory where she feels helpless. Her subconscious takes her to age seventeen where she is trying to get into equestrian school. When her application is denied multiple times, she once again feels that helplessness and frustration.

In our sessions, Tamara uncovers several deep-seated beliefs that sprung forth from these experiences. *"People don't trust or understand me. They ridicule my intelligence. They cannot see what I am capable of."* These beliefs fuel a distrust in authority figures, so she makes a commitment to herself, "*I will keep things within*." After this, she consistently buries her feelings, fails to stand up for herself, and remains forever watchful for that authority figure who might be able to exert their influence. Ultimately, these emotions all add up to one thing - she is literally angry at the whole wide world.

She comes to see that her anger and distrust informs her life in so many ways. Though she is highly capable and can do her work easily, her inability to get along well with others keeps holding her back in her job. Her personal relationships are lacking, too - she has been married more than once, she fights frequently with her current husband, and she has trouble creating long-lasting social friendships. Finally, it is making her physically sick. Tamara now sees that her social and physical problems are all tied to these beliefs generated from her experiences as a child and young adult. After our third appointment, she says, "*I feel halfway there,*" in terms of completely healing both her body and her mind.

In our next meeting, we further work to dissipate her negative emotions. This time she just sobs. She is finally able to acknowledge how devastating it was for her when she didn't get into equestrian school. "*I never grieved the loss of my dream.*" It takes her a long while during this session to find a place of acceptance and peace around this event.

In retrospect, in this session I actually witness Tamara moving through the Kübler-Ross Five Stages of Grief model (denial, anger, depression, bargaining, acceptance). Until now, she has been stuck in the anger stage, off and on touching depression; but this time, in the confine of her subconscious mind going through the session, she successfully moves through all the stages fully to reach acceptance in just over an hour! At the end of this fourth session, Tamara says, with relief noticeable in her voice, "*I found closure and now there is a sense of peace.*"

THE OUTCOME

That was my last session with her, but I have had the pleasure of talking with her periodically since then. She tells me she is now a completely different person, even concerning issues that we didn't actually touch on in session. She can now eat anything without symptoms; she has lost weight; her marriage has drastically improved; and she was surprised to be promoted in a relatively new job. In Tamara's own words:

> *"I am now living the life I want. I sometimes don't recognize the person I have become as myself. I feel I fit inside my skin for the first time in my memory. I go through my day calmly and with no stress - which is a totally new experience for me."*

Grief is powerful. We know that. Yet to realize that someone can stay stuck in one stage of loss for forty years... Well, I am still in awe of this! Tamara's case showcases that time does not necessarily heal all wounds.

What would have happened if Tamara had come to me as a doctor, rather than a hypnotherapist? It's a telling question. I know I would have followed medical guidelines, run my diagnostics, and prescribed medication; but just like the other medical professionals she had seen, it likely wouldn't have worked out for her. She wasn't content to take medications. Even so, because her emotions, sense of self, and disease states were all interconnected, I was never going to really help her with anything other than a holistic mode of healing.

Tamara's case helped me to see those patients that don't have a typical resolution to treatment in a completely different light. I experienced many of these patients who, after spending years in and out of the medical system for the same problem, radiated this "*you can't fix me*" attitude that was *forceful*. They would list all the diagnostics and medications they had tried and seemed almost whiny as they told me they weren't feeling any better. Sometimes they got labeled as "difficult" or "hypochondriacal." I understand that they don't have that point of view out of arrogance or inherent negativity; it's just that the medical system has repeatedly failed them. All they want is to feel better, but they have come away disappointed over and over again. So, they doctor-hop, hoping to find that one person who will both listen to and fix them, even as develop an attitude of defensiveness along the way because the doctors fail to see that it's not just the physical, but the emotional side as well, that needs healing.

Since emotion is energy in motion, each emotion we experience vibrates at its own frequency. For example, anger has one frequency and sadness another. In fact, our body's organs and systems have their own frequency, too, which means that energy from a particular emotion gets stored in the organ that most closely matches that frequency. There is evidence that suggests clear connections between specific emotions and areas of the body; for example, anger typically gets stored in the stomach, anxiety in your gut or intestine, and grief in your lungs. If doctors can begin to ask their patients targeted questions based on this information, I believe we will never see our patients or chronic illness the same way again.

Hypnotherapy opened me up to the power of asking some well-placed questions. “What is happening in your life now?” “What was happening in your life when this symptom first started?” “How are your relationships?” “Have you ever experienced any kind of trauma?” “How are you treated at work?” When you ask patients these kinds of questions you will inevitably get something like, “That’s when my mom passed away,” or “That’s when we declared bankruptcy." Listening and empathizing doesn’t take a college degree - and very often, a question asked with legitimate care and concern can lead patients to find their own answers.

Whenever a patient presents with seemingly intractable issues, I now work with the understanding that there is an emotional hook at the center - something in their past that is getting replayed in their current life. When we help them make this connection between their life experiences and their bodies it can yield amazing results. There is almost always something your patient can pinpoint that was going on when their symptoms started. This simple thing can potentially move them out of neutral - and even if it doesn’t, they feel seen and heard in a whole new way. There is no downside.

Medicine teaches doctors to identify patients by their disease and trains us to give prescriptions based on the physiology of that disease. But that didn't work with Tamara. Discovering that her emotions, her body, her life experiences, and her physical state were all connected was a revalidation of what I had learned during my hypnotherapy training. *This knowing completes me as a physician.*

> *"Taking a purely physiological approach to medicine can't work for everyone."*

CHAPTER TWELVE

SONIA: DARK AND LIGHT

"It was so palpable - the deep contrast between joy and sadness, helplessness and happiness, dancing and pain."

My first internship was in the gynecology department at a renowned hospital in Delhi. Just after I started, my mom found a lump in her abdomen, so I took her to my consultant to do an ultrasound. They found a cyst that was carcinogenic. Fortunately, she was Stage One; but they still recommended surgery, chemo, the whole works. Everything collapsed for me the day when she was diagnosed. I had never even seen my mom sick - not a cough, not a flu, nothing. Other than my patients, I had never really seen sickness up close and personal.

At that moment I became my mom's shadow, and my hospital became our whole world. Fortunately, I could keep my residency and shift my schedule when I needed to be with her. Each time she had chemo, surgery, or testing done, I was there. I was in such a haze. I have no recollection as to who was taking care of my dad or sisters, who was doing the cooking and cleaning. I was just so focused on my mother.

Soon after her first chemo, she ran her fingers through her wet hair after a bath - and a pile of it just fell out into her hand. I was there, and we exchanged that utter look of shock mixed with the pain of sensing what was coming ahead... No words were spoken, and yet so much was exchanged between us in that moment. We were both so devastated, and through our tears we knew that we both grieved something. I think we were mourning the loss of the innocence of life; we both knew life will not be the same after this. That moment is seared into my memory as one of the most heartbreaking, tender, and intimate of my life.

Later on, while working on myself during a practice session, my subconscious took me back in time to the same moment. I realized there was another exchange that took place that day that had implications for me down the line. When I took her hand that day, I gave her all my strength, sending it out in waves from my heart and my soul. And as I shared my positivity, love, and power with her, I (unknowingly) took on her helplessness. This transfer of emotions and energies, something we humans do fairly often without even being aware of it, would happen again later between my dad and myself.

* * * *

During my mom's first cancer diagnosis, she was hospitalized for most of her treatment. At one point after chemo, her hemoglobin dropped low enough to require a transfusion. I was an intern working under an assigned consultant, so I informed my consultant and asked for permission to transfuse, which I documented in my mom's file. My mistake, being a newbie in the world of hierarchical medicine, was not running this by the head of the department. Later, I realized that the department head and my consultant didn't get along; I was just a doctor and a daughter, trying to take care of my mom.

I could never have imagined my mom having a transfusion reaction - which obviously led the nurses to inform the head of the department, who literally came raging into my mom's room the next day and - in front of my mom – pronounced that I could have killed her! She condemned me as totally irresponsible to make the transfusion without the senior's consent. She didn't give me a chance to explain that I actually *did* get permission over the phone and documented it in the file. She kept demeaning me in front of my mother. I started to cry, and the helplessness I felt in that moment crushed my self-worth.

The next day, still upset and with teary eyes, I spoke to my ever even-keeled dad. To his credit, he didn't weigh in; he just let me work my way through it. Ultimately, I felt that, as a new doctor, I should perhaps apologize to the department head to clear the air between us. When I arrived at her office, she was with two other senior doctors. When she saw me, in front of the other two, she again accused me of not getting appropriate permission for a transfusion that could have caused irreversible harm. She then said the worst words any doctor can hear: "*I don't know how she is a doctor; she is going to kill someone. You don't deserve to be here.*" I was devastated at being shamed in front of the others. Without saying a word I ran out of her room, crying.

My dad saved my medical career that day. After being shamed and bullied in front of the seniors, I could have decided to leave medicine for good; or, I could have come out of that episode as a scarred young doctor. But my dad's response changed the worst possible scenario in an instant. He decided to remove my mom from that hospital against medical advice. He completely believed in me and the rightness of my actions. "*We will take her to another hospital - and if this decision brings anything back on you, we will file a case against your department head.*" God, what strength he gave me that day! He single-handedly gave me the gift of believing in myself, of standing up for myself, and not giving anyone else the power to crush my dreams or my worth.

It all turned out all right, eventually. We did go LAMA (Leaving Against Medical Advice) and I documented the reason why on my mom's medical file. Soon, it was the talk of the hospital - that an intern's mother left against medical advice because of the department head's behavior! Gradually the furor died away without any repercussions.

Looking back on this experience, I saw it was a mirror opposite to the one I shared with my mom when her hair started to fall out post-chemo. Back then, I took on her helplessness and gave her my strength; but here, in this moment of controversy, my dad took on my helplessness and gave me his strength.

Sometimes when we face hard times it is enough to hold someone's hand or vent out our feelings to a colleague, friend, spouse, or teacher. Sometimes when we are hurting we can get enough positive energies from outside ourselves to get us through. Yet, there are other experiences we keep to ourselves because of fear, vulnerability, or just an unawareness that these moments have had an impact. Only later did I realize that I kept most of those feelings and experiences to myself - and they left me holding onto some darkness that would surface later on.

* * * *

As mom's treatment ended, she was in remission. My residency ended shortly after that, and I was looking for a job. I applied to a lot of different positions - and as luck would have it, I was offered a position at the best cancer hospital in Delhi. Given the prestige of the post, it was hard to turn down. After a stint in the ICU at that hospital, I got shifted to the medical team in charge of cancer treatment for diagnosed patients, working for the best oncologist in the city.

Shortly thereafter, my mom's first annual post-treatment check-up came due. The scans found a new 0.22 centimeter lymph node in her pelvic area that looked cancerous. As the consultant broke this news to me, past memories of that painful journey flashed in front of my eyes. The thought that we had to watch her go through the whole thing once more... All that pain and discomfort, just about broke me... The same journey again... NO!

I went home that day not knowing how to break the news to her and to the rest of the family. Eventually, I found the courage to tell her that she had to repeat surgery and chemo all over again. I salute this woman who is my mother, that woman has the strength of a tiger! She cried briefly. Then she went to her hairdresser, chopped her gorgeous hair off, came back and said, *"Let's do this. I am ready."*

During this second round, post-chemo, she experienced terrible cramps and pain in her legs. I could see how much she was hurting, but I couldn't do anything to make her feel better. Medicines were not helping. As I sat by her feet, pressing her legs to make her feel better, I became aware of a wedding procession outside on the road. Weddings in India are high-energy affairs with drum rolls, happy music, and singing. Looking down from the darkness of my mom's second floor room, feeling my own helplessness and sadness, it was so palpable - the deep contrast between joy and sadness, helplessness and happiness, dancing and pain. To experience the duality in that moment was a deep awakening.

CHAPTER TWELVE

* * * *

The world we live in is that of duality. We can't know light without experiencing the dark, but we often forget this. That night in India, listening to the wedding procession, I saw the stark contrast between my sadness and their joy - and it gave me *hope*. Hope that my family, always a happy one before my mom's cancer, would get back there once again. Whoever said "*hope springs eternal*" was exactly right. It has to be, or nothing we humans do makes sense.

In order to be our most joyful, capable, authentic selves we must sometimes do the work of exploring our own negative emotions, mistakes, memories, experiences, and vulnerabilities. In my own hypnotherapy sessions, as I processed all of these moments in my life, I understood how they created that stress of taking on more responsibility as a doctor, friend, or wife than was actually mine. I understood the impact of the negative emotions of shame, humiliation, and helplessness that manifested in various parts of my life. Only when I explored that darkness within could I discover the light of my true self.

The practice of hypnotherapy is a brilliant bridge between our own darkness and light. Simply forgetting or sublimating our negative emotions and memories is a coping mechanism that will still result in "Dis-ease." Instead, hypnotherapy brings our emotions back into balance by flipping the negative to the positive while still allowing us to retain the memory.

"Our subconscious is
our greatest resource precisely because
it contains all opposites and, in their
reunion, we become whole."

CHAPTER THIRTEEN

KARINA: TROUBLE LETTING GO

"I want the doctor who is doing things differently."

THE PROBLEM

I met Karina in Dubai. I had just started integrating hypnotherapy into my medical practice and she happened to hear me that day I did the radio show. She couldn't wait to book an appointment. When she called, she told my staff, "*I want the doctor who is doing things differently.*"

Karina is petite, delicate, and appears both sophisticated and artsy. There is a depth to her - she is *soulful*, both in the way she expresses herself and the feeling that you get when you are in her presence. She came to me because she had been suffering from chronic constipation. It began after she had undergone four surgeries within two years: one for intestinal obstruction; the next for post-op peritonitis; then, an umbilical hernia repair; and finally, a repeat hernia repair two months after the first. She said the constipation began after these surgeries.

Like many of my patients, Karina was disappointed with the limitations of mainstream medicine. None of the doctors she saw had found a reason for the constipation. Every colonoscopy, CT scan with contrast, and MRI came back clean. In addition, she practiced a healthy vegan diet, exercised regularly, ate extra fiber, didn't smoke or imbibe alcohol, drank quite a lot of water, and had cut out all processed foods. Her constipation didn't make sense from a medical standpoint. Though her doctors assured her there was nothing physically wrong with her, she only had one or two bowel movements a week. To Karina, her constipation was very, very real.

She told me that she had always felt "*dirty from the inside,*" and was often irritable because of this feeling. After a while, this led to OCD-like behavior focused around constant thoughts that she was unclean. She began taking showers two or three times a day and drinking a lot of water to soothe herself. To her credit, she recognized that there was an emotional component to her constipation, and that she was headed in a bad direction.

CHAPTER THIRTEEN

THE SESSIONS

Karina's sessions focused on emotions of guilt and grief anchored in her childhood. She was the result of an unplanned pregnancy, conceived before her parents were married. She understood all of this indirectly. Like so many families, no one ever explicitly told her she was unplanned; it was *in the air*. But that feeling of being unwanted had a direct impact on her self-worth.

In addition, her father was physically abusive to her mother for as long as Karina could remember. Every time she witnessed her dad beating her mom, this feeling that she should be able to save her mom welled up - followed by grief at being helpless to do so. This initiated a pattern of feeling guilty for things that were outside of her control. Though her dad never abused her, Karina's childhood was filled with tension, fear, and uncertainty. She recalls never feeling happy or truly cared for by her parents.

What we first uncovered in session was that, underneath her guilt, there was a great deal of hidden anger towards her mom. In trance, seeing herself as a young girl, she hurled questions at her mom with great force - "*Why are you letting him do this to you?*" "*Why can't you just leave him and be free?*" As she released this anger, she experienced profound sadness because she was never able to just be a kid: to be happy, spontaneous, or free.

We also discovered that, though her dad never raised a hand towards her, he was super analytical and critical. Karina was constantly on guard because he analyzed everything. Nothing she ever did was good enough. This had lasting effects on her self-esteem and life choices. While Karina was aware that she had a artistic flair - she loved to write and always felt like she could be successful doing it - she would kill any writing effort as soon as it began because her dad's legacy of criticism and abuse left her with two main beliefs: "*I'm not allowed to be happy,*" and, "*It won't be good enough.*" This stifled her creativity and joy.

In our sessions we also explored loss after loss after loss. Karina was close to her grandmother, who gave her some of the love she didn't get at home. Her grandma died of cancer when Karina was a young woman; Karina was unable to see her before she passed, creating guilt and sadness that she had never fully processed. That same year, Karina's mom was diagnosed with breast cancer. She went into remission with treatment, but had a recurrence two years after Karina got married. Around the same time, Karina's husband of two years died in a car accident. Unbelievably, the losses didn't stop there. Her mom then had a third relapse and died. Her mother-in-law, whom she was also close to, died suddenly of a brain hemorrhage. In every instance, Karina felt "not enough"- that she should have done more. She had become mired in a relentless cycle of guilt and grief, grief and guilt.

Karina had been holding on to these huge energies in her body for a long time – sadness over her lost childhood and over all those people close to her who had died. With every loss she experienced, she somehow felt she was to blame. Her running theme was, "*If I had done more, this wouldn't have happened.*" Because she was so focused on her own culpability, she never really allowed herself to grieve.

I did three sessions with Karina. In each one, she subconsciously released layer after layer of emotions. Most of all, she rewired that running tape of guilt that would not allow her to let go of the grief... almost like a self-punishment. Reviewing the entire journey retrospectively, Karina was able to forgive herself with a knowing that she actually *was* enough and *did* enough. That was the inner shift that resolved her physical problems!

THE OUTCOME

The email I received from her a couple of weeks later was so amazing. She wrote that after two weeks her constipation was gone. She felt free. "*I can finally let go with ease.*"

What is constipation, really? From a medical standpoint, it is defined as infrequent bowel movements (less than three times per week) or the difficult passage of stool. But from an energetic standpoint, it is *an inability to let go*. Karina was literally holding on to emotions - blame, guilt, anger, sadness, and an inability to love herself

- so tightly that her body had no choice but to respond with a holding on of its own. And, as she dispersed those dense, heavy emotions, she flowed.

Loss is a recurring theme in my hypnotherapy practice. We don't do well in today's world with death. We don't talk about it, process it, or even accept it as a natural part of life. As a result, death is often a trigger. In Karina's case, her tipping point of disease started after the death of her beloved mother-in-law. Everyone she tried to hold on to left, in one way or another; and each loss was encased in guilt and self-blame. In fact, Karina's numerous surgeries showcased the body's breakdown and its inability to handle the energy of all the undigested emotions from the past. Not surprisingly, post-surgery constipation popped up because she still hadn't dealt with the underlying cause of her "*Dis*-ease." After an abdominal surgery, doctors often blame post-surgical adhesions as the reason for any disturbance in the gut - but there is often more to it, and Karina's resolution of symptoms proves that.

"We humans often become frustrated and angry at illness, but it's time we begin to understand that illness can be our best clue to what (really) ails us."

Karina's case confirmed that whenever there is a patient with unresolved physical issues, it is time to start asking targeted questions about their life experiences.

When we begin to look at chronic illness in this light, both as doctors and as patients, then I believe we will see changes in the way we deliver healthcare that will lead to improved health and wellness.

"Where and how our bodies manifest disease can lead us to specific emotions that need to be released."

CHAPTER FOURTEEN

SONIA: LESSONS

"Not being good enough."

Like many of us, I know the feeling of not being good enough. I am fortunate that I was able to uncover these unconscious beliefs that manifested in a sense of over-attachment to my patients. I constantly wondered, "Have I done enough?" I would come home after a day at the clinic or the hospital, still ruminating over a particular patient. My very practical spouse would just look at me, shake his head, and say something like, "*Don't you see this type of patient every day? Why are you so worked up over this?*" Frankly, I never had a good answer.

It was years later that I realized that my subconscious thoughts had led to an unhealthy level of stress that was over and above the rigors of daily practice. I suspect I am not alone in this. This took me a while to unpack, but through my own hypnotherapy sessions, I uncovered that my sense of not being good enough collided with guilt during a few pivotal moments when my personal and professional lives intersected.

While living in Singapore, I moved from pediatrics into geriatrics and fell in love with this population. One of the biggest downsides, though, was seeing the way we used medications that (at times) didn't seem to be in their best interest. I saw so many elderly patients on a cocktail of medications that chemically didn't agree with each other - often resulting in new symptoms which needed further medications. The result was a general malaise, even a stupor, in many of them. In addition, I frequently experienced confused patients restrained in a hospital setting. This disturbed me internally, generating a sense of guilt. I just knew that restraining patients was wrong and that there had to be another way, but I didn't know what. At a later stage in my career, my staff nurses knew that when I was on rounds, my patients should not be on restraints - it was an order. I do appreciate the limitations of our current system that makes restraints practical (being short-staffed, the litigiousness of our society, etc.). But for me, it came down to a personal choice: I no longer wanted to be a part of the cause of so much suffering when I had taken an oath to alleviate it.

Later, when I was able to look at my feelings around this, I understood that it stemmed from my desire to treat all patients as human beings deserving of love, compassion, and healing. My inner guilt was leading me on a journey - one that looked for ways to change how I practiced within our current system to reflect this inner knowing.

Within a few years after my mom's second bout with cancer, my sister and I both got married; we moved away to different countries, while my youngest sister was still at home. I relocated to Singapore and then to Dubai. Both were a short flight home, but felt like an ocean's worth of time and space.

I still talked to my mom by phone all the time. One day she mentioned to me that she was feeling depressed. This was likely due to the chemotherapy drugs that saved her life but also damaged that delicate biochemical balance, the microbiome, in her gut and brain. With some effort, I got her in to see a psychiatrist - who immediately started her on antidepressants. But these didn't have the desired effect. Instead of lifting her mood, it turned her into a mere shadow of herself. Sleeping was the only thing she looked forward to. She had lost her joy, and regardless of tweaks in her medication, she just didn't perk up.

During one of our phone conversations, mom confessed she was having suicidal thoughts. I'll never forget the sentence she uttered: "*I just want to end it. I constantly think about ending my life.*"

Being the only medical professional in the family, I sprang into action once again. I instructed my dad and sister to never leave her alone - not even for a second. But as life would have it, one day my dad decided to go downstairs to get the mail at the same time that my sister left to go grocery shopping. Though my mom was only alone for the briefest of time, she was able to talk neighbors into giving her their key to the building's fifth-floor rooftop terrace. Despite months of antidepressant medication, my mom jumped.

Theoretically, a five-story fall is not survivable; and yet my mom did survive, with little more than a skull fracture, a lacerated nose, and two broken teeth. No broken bones, no internal bleeding. She landed on a parapet first, which slowed her momentum. Due to her head injury, she ended up in the ICU in an extremely agitated state.

She was in the hospital with a concussion, confused, and agitated. She couldn't be sedated as per the protocol for post head injury. My mom, not understanding why she was restrained, fought desperately to escape her restraints. Seeing this brought up those other times when I had seen my geriatric patients restrained and fighting, creating this loop of disorientation, agitation, restraint, then even more disorientation and agitation. I remember thinking that the more you restrain someone who can't process the reason for their confinement, the crazier they get.

Watching my own mom tied down did something to me, as both a daughter and a doctor. I was a like a roaring lion, telling the nurses to untie her! Getting nowhere, I took charge. I convinced them to take off the restraints and that I would calm her down. And, of course, once she was free and recognized that I was by her side, she settled down and was not agitated. She stayed calm throughout her stay in the hospital. All she needed was words of reassurance to calm her down - not restraints.

It took time after she came home, but Mom gradually came back to herself. The depression was still in the background, but she no longer had suicidal thoughts. To this day, she has no memory of getting that terrace key from the neighbor, jumping off that roof, or much of the aftermath. She finds it almost impossible to believe she tried to kill herself. "*Why would I do this*?" As if she was not herself when she decided to jump.

Her teeth were repaired, but her lacerated nose did not retain its original shape, despite three procedures with the best plastic surgeons. Whenever I looked at her nose, *I felt like a failure as a doctor*. Almost a year later, I confessed to my dad that I felt so guilty about everything that happened; perhaps I did not do enough when she told me about the suicidal thoughts. I carried that guilt within because I was unable to prevent her suicide attempt. My beautiful dad's amazing response was to see the bigger picture. "*There is a reason we had to experience all of this as a family, and an even bigger reason you experienced this as a doctor. You don't know what that is yet, but you will.*"

* * * *

My dad was right; there *was* a reason I had these experiences. I wouldn't wish for them; but collectively, they were supreme teaching moments.

When I did a deep dive into my subconscious mind during one of the mandatory practice sessions, I reviewed all of these snapshots in time. I understood that I can't stop bad things from happening (even if I am a doctor); that I am not omnipotent. With that understanding I was then able to shift guilt into learning invaluable lessons about myself and my life, pushing me into growth and change, with self-acceptance. This work helped me become a happier, more centered person and a better doctor.

As I reviewed this part of my life's journey subconsciously, as a doctor, I had a sense that medicine is, indeed, fallible. This was very unconscious to me back then as I unknowingly started seeking answers outside the field of mainstream medicine. And it was just a few short months after that conversation with my Dad that I heard about hypnotherapy training from a colleague. My life, the way I thought about health, and the way I chose to help people were all about to drastically change.

"The Doctor was turning into a Healer."

CHAPTER FIFTEEN

EVE: SWALLOWING SADNESS

"You are free to be the child."

THE PROBLEM

Eve is a tall, striking woman with a smile that projects her good-hearted nature. She is highly empathetic. She is always ready to help anyone and everyone - frequently shedding her own tears whenever she talks about the pain of someone else. I met her in a hypnotherapy training I was conducting. As a student, she soon realized that she had her own healing to do, so she booked an appointment.

Her presenting issue was a persistent lump in her throat. She first noticed that sensation three years prior. She had trouble swallowing, especially when she turned her head to one side. The lump wasn't painful, just annoying. Though she could not feel any lump to touch, she could clearly feel its presence.

Eve saw her general practitioner who referred her to an ENT. A laryngeal scope and ultrasound were ordered and the results were negative. An MRI was scheduled but not yet completed when she found herself telling her friend about this weird sensation. The friend happened to be familiar with a condition called *globus pharynges*; after hearing it described, Eve was sure that this was what was wrong with her.

Eve had none of the underlying medical or psychological conditions that typically cause globus - GERD, anxiety, depression, esophagitis, or a musculoskeletal condition. What she did have was a sudden onset of stress right before her symptoms started. Eve's stressor had to do with her brother, who had a terrible fight with his wife. He called her at midnight one night, frantic, to ask for her help. The police were called, there was loads of drama, and she didn't sleep for about thirty hours straight. As Eve is typically the person in her family of origin who "*sorts everything out*" for everyone else, her stress in those thirty hours was overwhelming. It was only a few days later that she first felt the lump.

Unfortunately, though she believed she understood the cause, the globus sensation persisted. It had abated somewhat over the previous three years, but just before she met with me, the sensation had come back with a vengeance. There also wasn't much she could do to relieve her symptoms. "*The only thing my doctors offered was to take antacids, but I knew this wasn't the solution because it has never helped.*"

CHAPTER FIFTEEN

THE SESSIONS

As we began our first session, I asked Eve to get in touch with that sensation in her throat and to visualize what it might represent. As she deepened in trance, her husband immediately came to mind. She had been worried about his health because he had recently had a bout with cancer; although it was in remission, she had noticed some physical changes in him that made her worry. Of course, she had expressed her concerns to him, but he wouldn't talk about it, so she kept most of her worries to herself. She began to cry, saying, "*I don't want to be alone. I love him and I am scared to lose him. I am scared of not being loved.*" As she voiced it, I thought her fear of not being loved was interesting; the Pandora box was opening. So, I asked Eve to see that younger part of herself who was afraid of not being loved and that initiated a cascade of memories.

As we got in touch with all of the times that she felt scared, uncomfortable, alone, and not loved, Eve came in touch with her four-year-old self, yearning for her dad's presence, as her dad was not really around when she was a child. She wanted him to be there much more often than he was because she loved and counted on him. During our session she was able to express this to her father in the confines of her mind, and she felt her dad responded by saying, "*I am so sorry. I thought you knew how much I loved you. I thought I was giving you everything you needed.*" In that moment as an adult, Eve realized that her dad had his own struggles as a man, and that those struggles might have kept him from being fully present. This beautiful conversation between the adult, child, and father ended with Dad "holding" the four-year-old Eve in his arms, letting her fill up on all the love she had been longing for.

Eve then tapped into a sadness within her younger self that remained even after she made peace with her dad. This sadness had two origins. The first came from her parents constant fighting, which created feelings of uncertainty. The second stemmed from her mom, who was never in touch with Eve's emotions. Through back-and-forth dialogue with her mom in trance, Eve realized that her mom had so much going on within herself; and with five kids, she was never able to fully pay attention to each kid, making her seem emotionally unavailable. Suddenly, Eve understood why she was so insecure in her dad's absence. She had no choice but to keep these emotions within, almost trying to "gulp" them.

Finally, we uncovered the final link to Eve's globus. Her brother comes into her mind and she becomes aware that they shared the same sadness as children. He also experienced that same lack of parental attention that Eve did. Eve not only took on her own sadness, but she took on her brother's, too.

After working with Eve to process all of those undigested emotions, I ask her to let her inner child know that, "All your needs are going to be fulfilled by me, little one. I am there for you totally and completely. You are free to be the child. I will take over as the adult from here." And as this scene ends, almost like a saga, a drama with a happy ending, the adult and the child are embraced in a hug by their parents. Having let go of the sadness, they are now able to fill up completely with love. As we end the session, Eve has a distinct sense that her own energies of love, security, and fulfillment are coming back into her body. She sighs deeply.

THE OUTCOME

Afterwards, Eve became conscious of so many things she missed doing as a child - so much fun - because her parents weren't available to her. When I followed up with Eve about a month later, she told me that the sensation of the lump in her throat had started to dissipate within a few days of our session. It was completely gone in a couple of weeks.

"My throat has felt fully normal now for about two weeks! It is unique when I listen back on our session that my little self felt sad for her brother (I still do at times) so it really connected everything! Listening to our session again connected that in such a deep way; and with this awareness, I am able to understand my boundaries and priorities for myself much better."

Like so many of my other patients, Eve made other changes in her life, too. She quit her job shortly after working with me, saying, "*I am ready for a new chapter.*" She is now fully immersed in learning the modality that changed her life for better.

Eve literally was unable to swallow her sadness. Though Eve wouldn't have fallen seriously ill from globus, her body was clearly calling out to her, asking her to pay attention to long-buried emotions.

As a doctor, it blew my mind to see these different facets of disease and to validate that what really ails us is our emotions. It seems so unrealistic if you only see it from a scientific perspective. But Eve's case is a great example of how an outward, physical symptom can be an accurate interpretation of an internal struggle. We've all heard (and probably used) expressions such as "broken heart," "pounding headache," and yes, a "lump in the throat." These idioms exists because they truthfully portray how an emotion can manifest in our physiology.

"As a doctor, I couldn't be of much help; but as a hypnotherapist, I had an impact."

CHAPTER SIXTEEN

SONIA: SHARED JOURNEYS ARE THE BEST JOURNEYS

"When we, as doctors, reclaim our own power, we can help our patients reclaim theirs."

I've admitted to being pretty entangled with my patients. For me, it was more than just the pure desire of being a doctor. It was about taking 100% responsibility for the success or failure of my patients. I know that's not a healthy goal; it's a stressor.

Looking back, I realized that if I had a patient who wasn't getting well, I would be calling to check on them, Googling, looking at research articles, and calling other doctors. I was thinking about my patients when I was at home and at work. After a while, it felt like I was literally breathing for them. And it was always *my* failure, never theirs. Then I would often lose my cool with nurses and other providers when they didn't live up to my over-the-top expectations. I was going off-balance.

Rather than looking at this dispassionately, I just thought I had to dig in more. I had to work harder. But working harder isn't the best answer because lack of rest and self-care has consequences. It finally started to niggle at me that I was incomplete as a doctor - incomplete in my power to heal.

We were taught in med school that our patients have some control over their health, but never that they have an ability to impact their own *healing*. Why is it that we believe they have agency over one but not the other? Try as I might, I can't be, nor should I be, 100% responsible for their wellness. It took doing my own work, releasing emotions of guilt and over-responsibility, for me to understand that I am on a shared journey with my patients. We are in it together. This total partnership with my patients is a side benefit of hypnotherapy that I didn't expect.

As a hypnotherapist, I become the GPS, but the patient is always the driver and that's a partnership which yields amazing results. Knowing their life stories helps me to road map the subconscious and navigate them to those specific moments from the past which are responsible for creating the "Dis-ease" in the present. But for me to take up the role of the navigator, the patient has to take the responsibility to drive - and be willing to go to those junctions back in time which are either forgotten or buried deep within.

As a hypnotherapist, it has been proven to me that my patients have a deep well of inner resources to draw from. Now that I know this, I have a choice. I can reinforce the standard belief, supported by modern medicine, that something out there caused the problem; or...

"I CAN CREATE
A NEW PARADIGM
THAT AT ITS CORE SAYS,
'IF YOU HAVE A
PROBLEM, YOU
SOMEWHERE HAVE
CREATED IT -
AND YOU, YOURSELF,
CAN RESOLVE IT.'"

CHAPTER SEVENTEEN

CIGARETTES: MAN'S BEST FRIEND?

"I will never touch cigarettes again. I am a different man altogether."

THE PROBLEM

Smoking is preventable, and yet it is a leading cause of death throughout the world. It's also something I really struggled with in my practice. Like many other doctors, I just wasn't having much success at getting my patients to quit smoking. The pull of cigarettes was much stronger than the notion that at some point in time they might get sick. In addition to counseling them on the risks every chance I got, I offered nicotine replacement and other pharmacologic approaches. Even so, most would relapse within a fairly short period of time.

I wasn't the only one struggling. Typically, physician intervention works in less than 5% of patients; and this low statistic doesn't take relapse into account. Treating smoking addiction was discouraging to say the least - and it led me to consider other tools that would allow me to meet the needs of my patients.

We tend to put smokers into one, all-encompassing bracket; but I no longer believe that's an accurate representation of smoking addiction. For some, habit is at the crux of why they smoke; but for others, unprocessed trauma and emotion are at the core. As you read these case studies, you'll see that while the circumstances surrounding their smoking differ, the treatment is essentially the same: Revisit the trauma, release the emotion, and thereby erase the need for cigarettes. It sounds simple - and ultimately, it is.

You probably won't believe me, but when I began using hypnotherapy with my smokers, I started getting unprecedented results - to the tune of a 95% success rate. It was nothing short of amazing. Not only that, but these patients rarely returned to smoking. The work isn't easy. It generally takes intense sixty- to ninety-minute sessions, delivered every day for five days in a row, to be effective; but it is so incredibly worth it.

Over the last three years I have worked with dozens of smokers and have learned some things about this tough-to-beat addiction. First, this population can be broken into two types. One is the "identification" smoker. This person typically picks up the habit as a way of identifying with their peers. They aren't all that attached to cigarettes; it's more about belonging in a social situation than any kind of need. Identification smokers can quit pretty easily, even if it entails going "cold turkey," once they make up their minds to do it. They don't actually need hypnotherapy or other interventions; willpower usually does the trick.

The second, and much more intractable type, is the "replacement" smoker. This person smokes as a way to cope with loss, often finding cigarettes by accident during a traumatic event, such as a divorce, breakup, or death of a loved one. When they are stressed and anxious, smoking helps them to fill a void and replace their sense of calm and clarity. Quitting for this type of smoker is much more difficult; even if they can manage it, relapse rates are high.

I found these replacement smokers to be well-educated, highly responsible people who tend to internalize their emotions. They understand the health risks to themselves and the harms of passive smoking on their families. They are acutely aware that their addiction is illogical - yet they cannot quit. This mystifies them as much as it does their family and friends. By the time I meet them, replacement smokers have quit many times, only to resume a few months or even years later. When I ask them why they relapse, they almost always refer to some stressful thing that happened in their lives and say, *"I just needed a cigarette."* They will literally tell me that cigarettes have become their best friend.

The most telling commonality I found in all replacement smokers is an experience in childhood, usually between the ages of eight and fourteen, that brought a lot of stress and anxiety. The end result is a feeling of over-responsibility and of not being good enough. They don't start smoking then; it's later on, in early adulthood or later years, that another experience occurs which mimics the stress of their childhood. It's at this moment that someone else notices their anxiety and introduces them to smoking as a way to help them calm down. Once they experience that first deep, centering inhale followed by the dopamine-filled calm and clarity of the nicotine, they are hooked. In this cohort, I have always uncovered a childhood experience that is at the root of their addiction. That's why these smokers require different tools.

The four cases in this chapter are a snapshot of the many replacement smokers I have worked with. They all smoked a pack to two packs a day for over a decade. Every one of them quit smoking, without relapse, after our sessions.

THE SESSIONS: NORMAN

"Why did you leave me?"

Norman, in his early forties, is both masculine and sophisticated. He is exceedingly articulate, charming, with impeccable manners. He has smoked more than a pack a day for over twenty years.

When Norman was thirteen, his dad died of a heart attack, leaving his mom alone to raise him and his little sister. Before his dad's death, he had a storybook life. His mom was a homemaker, the family was relatively well-off, and he could just be a kid without a lot of pressure. When his dad died, Norman became the man of the house overnight and the family struggled for money. "*I used to look at other kids who had things that were for fun or entertainment and I would think 'No, I have a mother and a sister to take care of. I can't indulge in anything fun.'*"

The responsibility was overwhelming; and with it came a lot of anxiety. "*What if I can't put food on the table? What if I can't keep everyone safe? What if I fail in my exams and I can't get a job?*" Though his mom was doing everything in her power to bring in income, and she never implied that Norman was in any way responsible for their well-being, both his culture and his own sense of family created that stress and pressure. He went from a secure, carefree kid to one who was anxious, uncertain, and stressed out. He could never relax.

Norman was able to go to university with the help of extended family and graduated at the age of 21. After graduation he lived with these extended family members in a large city and looked for his first job. After some time beating the pavement, he still had no offers. Now the anxiety that had been his constant companion since the age of 13 kicked into overdrive. This was especially true as his sister was now college age and needed money for her continued education.

In our first session, Norman clearly recalled the moment when he became a smoker. One evening the restlessness, pressure, and anxiety were at an all-time high; so much so that he went out for a walk to calm down. Suddenly, he smelled a cigarette; and right away he had the feeling that everything was going to be all right. He bought his first pack of cigarettes that night. When he took that first drag, he felt clear-headed and secure.

The huge realization for Norman in this session was that cigarettes were his connection to his dad, who also used to smoke. When he smelled that first cigarette and felt that everything was going to be O.K., the powerful memory of his dad - that person who always took care of his family - became anchored in him at that moment. His dad was the epitome of solidness and safety, and this is the emotional connection that Norman linked to smoking.

Understanding this changed everything for him. This alpha male cried like a baby when he understood that cigarettes were a representation of his dad. Norman realized that if he quit smoking, it would be like letting go of Dad all over again. Cigarettes linked him back to that feeling he had before the age of 13 - that life was safe and certain.

In his multiple sessions, I guided Norman to find closure with his dad's death. In trance, that 13-year-old part of him cried his heart out, begging to know, "*Why did you leave me*?" His grief mixed with anger and exhaustion from being that over-responsible kid who was now a man was heart-wrenching. As he expressed all of these emotions to his dad, his dad's response was, "*I'm so proud of you. You have done so well. You are fantastic.*" It dawned on Norman that he had never heard any adult tell him that he was enough, that he had succeeded. He had no idea how hungry he was for this validation.

Norman saw that he had never stopped to rest or relax since his dad's death, nor was he able to acknowledge, or enjoy, his own victories. His stress and anxiety just continued to pile up. In our final two sessions, he was able to acknowledge all of his successes - running his own company, employing 100 people, putting food on the table, having a wife and two kids. He finally recognized that his life was a blessing.

In our final session, he brought his cigarettes and lighter with him and threw them in the trash can.

He has never smoked again. He knew he was enough.

THE SESSIONS: TANESH

"Raised to be civilized at all costs"

Tanesh is in his early forties and quiet. He speaks only when spoken to, and his responses are tailored and straightforward. The man just doesn't indulge in chitchat. He had smoked a pack a day for the last ten years and was very conscious about how much he smoked. "*If I'm not paying attention, I could easily smoke two packs - but I make sure I stop at one.*"

Tanesh knew beyond a doubt that smoking was bad for him, and he had tried to quit many times. After ten years of a pack-a-day habit, he could tell his stamina was affected. He also knew his family hated his smoking. His elderly parents never said a word, but it was clear through their body language and facial expressions that they didn't like it. His wife, on the other hand, was much more vocal. He was also concerned because he had a young son and worried that he would grow up without a dad someday. After a decade of smoking, he was looking for a way to quit smoking once and for all.

Tanesh grew up in a small nuclear family with his parents and younger brother. His parents weren't talkative, but they lived by a highly structured code of right and wrong. This meant that Tanesh was always on high alert, having to sense whether he was doing the right thing through their facial expressions and body language. Emotions were never discussed. There was also a lot of importance placed on how the family was perceived by others, adding to the pressure of trying to get it right in the absence of spoken rules. Though his childhood was free from trauma or abuse, there was a sense of anxiety caused by never knowing exactly where he stood.

Tanesh was the oldest child. From the beginning, he felt responsible for his younger brother, who often looked to him as a role model. This made Tanesh feel that if he did something wrong, his brother would also suffer the repercussions.

At the age of 14, Tanesh was sent to boarding school. In this new environment, the unsaid message from his parents was that he must perform well, make them proud, and help keep their status within the community. Once again, this was unwritten and unspoken; but nonetheless, it was *loud.*

In his first appointment, Tanesh put all the pieces together regarding his family life. He understood for the first time that he always felt he was on "*shaky ground*" growing up. Decisions were made for him by his parents, plus all of the unspoken rules that, when broken, garnered a swift response. Even as an adult, he constantly worried that he wasn't good enough or wasn't making the right decisions. This uncertainty led him to procrastinate, which caused even more stress.

In our sessions, Tanesh explored his sadness around the fact that his parents never praised him or validated his accomplishments. One memory surfaced around bringing his report card home. He was so proud - he had scored a 98% - but his dad's only comment was, "*Why don't you have 100%*? Where did you lose the 2%?" The message was loud and clear: You must be perfect or you are not worthy.

At our next meeting, Tanesh witnessed in retrospect the exact moment when cigarettes came in to his life. Tanesh got married, and two years later his first child, a son, was born. The pregnancy was perfect - no complications - and his wife's labor was normal until, without warning, the baby went into distress. Suddenly, everyone around them started to move with urgency. As the attending OB was tied up with another emergency, it took a while to get Tanesh's wife into surgery. As the baby was removed during an emergency C-section, Tanesh could immediately see that his son was stillborn. The attempt to revive the baby was unsuccessful. Throughout this ordeal, the hospital staff communicated very little to them about what was happening, almost echoing childhood experiences of uncomfortable silence.

As he reviewed this traumatic life event in trance, Tanesh could feel his life literally stopped in that moment. He knew he was in shock and was able to sense all the thoughts that were running through his mind. "*How will I tell my wife?*" "*How am I supposed to handle this?*" "*How will she react?*" "*How do I support her when I can't handle my own emotions?*" "*Who is supposed to tell her: the doctor or me?*" He was utterly at a loss.

After a while, the doctors finally came in to talk to them - but they were devoid of any emotion or sympathy. Tanesh recalled that they just acted like this sort of thing happened all the time. It felt like another blow. At this moment in our session, his anger engulfed him.

"Why did they take so long to get her into surgery?" "The way they handled it was bullshit! It's all their fault that I lost my son!"

When Tanesh was finally able to leave his sedated wife so she could sleep, the first thing he found while walking out of the hospital was a cigarette. Someone was smoking just outside of the entrance, and Tanesh bummed a cigarette without even thinking. The feeling of that first inhale and how it calmed him down was so vivid. It was in this moment that he became a smoker.

In another session, Tanesh acknowledged that the death of the baby created a huge gap between him and his wife; yet they still wanted to have another child. Several years after their loss they were pregnant again. Devastatingly, at the eighteen-week mark, a Trisomy 18 test came back positive; they also discovered a hole in the baby's heart. Now they had to decide whether or not to bring this second baby into the world. The doctors told them that it would be very difficult to raise this child, and that the quality of life of the child would be poor. With a very heavy heart, they elected to not go through with the pregnancy.

As Tanesh reexamined this period in his life, he understood that the gap between him and his wife got even wider at this point, and it really started to take a toll. He also realized that cigarettes had become his best friend because they helped him deal with his inner anger and sadness.

His wife did become pregnant for a third time, and this baby was born healthy. Tanesh's son, who was now five years old, was his pride and joy; and yet, Tanesh could see that he wasn't really present for his living child. This piled on even more anxiety. He knew, deep down, that he wasn't doing enough for the son who was actually here. This further anchored his need to smoke.

In one of our final meetings, Tanesh saw that because he was raised to be "civilized" at all costs, he was never able to express his emotions in any of these traumatic circumstances. It was huge for him to understand that all of that unprocessed grief and anger led him to keep his distance from his wife and son. He was finally able to let go of all those heavy emotions.

In that same session, Tanesh was able to connect to his two unborn children. In trance, he was able to express his love for them, and these babies were able to share with him that no one did anything wrong; it just wasn't their time to be born yet. "*We don't want you to stay in the past. We are good where we are, and we sense your love.*" Afterwards, Tanesh said he could now simply feel connected to them without the baggage of all the sadness. Now his bond with these two babies was no longer about pain, but about love.

Three days after our last session, Tanesh said this...

CHAPTER SEVENTEEN

"It's out. I will never touch cigarettes again. I am a different man altogether."

THE SESSIONS: JOSEPH

"Am I self-sabotaging?"

Joseph is in his twenties. He is a marathon runner and a triathlete. He is fully conscious that it is ridiculous for him to be a high-level athlete and a smoker. "*Smoking is self-sabotaging to the max. Bloody hell, why am I doing this to myself?*" He had tried to quit many times and didn't get why he couldn't just walk away from something that was so bad for his health. It didn't make any sense.

Jospeh grew up the oldest of three, having one brother and one sister. His parents were divorced when he was 13; after that, he lived full-time with his mother. At the same time, he was coming to terms with the fact that he was gay, though he would keep this to himself until he turned 16.

In our first session, Joseph reviewed the memory that directly led to his smoking. He saw his mom and dad fighting, and it was clear that his dad had cheated on his mom. This was the reason for the divorce. The fight ended with his mom literally pushing his dad out of the house. At that moment, Joseph realized that he felt like he had to protect his mom because he could see how much pain she was in; he could see her vulnerability.

Until then Joseph's dad, a successful banker, had always brought home plenty of money and was the undisputed head of the household. Afterwards, his dad stopped being the provider for their family. Joseph went from a pretty easy childhood to one of struggle in an instant. As he randomly met his dad after the divorce, Joseph recognized that he and his dad never talked about any of this, including Joseph's constant fears that they wouldn't be able to survive economically. His dad, who was once his role model, was now a betrayer who brought pain and uncertainty into the family.

Throughout our sessions, Joseph discovered feelings of betrayal and anger that he had successfully repressed until now. He also saw many of his own relationships in a new light. It was a major realization to see the connection between his dad's betrayal and Joseph's frequent attraction to people who would ultimately come to betray him.

Joseph's first real homosexual relationship, when he was 17, was with a much older man who was addicted to drugs and alcohol. This was the person who introduced him to cigarettes and drugs, both of which helped Joseph cope with the stress and anxiety that became a part of his life after the parent's divorce. Joseph realized that both marathon running and smoking were ways to cope with these feelings. He also figured out that his self-sabotaging behaviors were a way of defying his dad. By harming himself, he was trying to show his dad, "*See you didn't do such a good job of raising me.*" Ironically, Joseph actually had no idea if his dad even cared that he smoked.

In a later session, Joseph saw that smoking merely kept him stuck in his old issue with authority that started with his parent's divorce. He was able to acknowledge that his mom and dad both remarried pretty happily - he was the only one who remained stuck in those old energies.

In trance, Joseph was able to confront his father and all the others who had betrayed and took advantage of him. Afterwards, he clearly saw a part of himself that was destroying his own life to prove some kind of point. As our final session ended, he threw away his cigarettes with ease.

At the six-month mark, Joseph felt a pull to return to smoking. He actually took one puff and it freaked him out, so he contacted me right away. I decided to teach Joseph self-hypnosis so that he could deal with any potential relapses on his own. By chance, I was giving a seminar to smokers on the benefits of hypnotherapy as a tool for smoking cessation, which included training in self-hypnosis; so I invited Joseph to learn with the group, and he agreed to attend.

As the presentation progressed, Jospeh saw that the group thought I was inflating my success and (I loved him so much for this) he stood up and said, "*I am a marathon runner and I used to smoke. This hypnotherapy stuff works. I am here today to vouch for this. I walked out of her office a nonsmoker. You should listen to her."* Joseph has been smoke-free ever since.

THE SESSIONS: CALLUM

"You are good for nothing!"

Callum, a man in his forties, had been smoking a pack a day for twenty years. The reason he gave himself and everyone else for smoking was: "*Too much stress at work.*"

In our first session, we found the root of Cal's addiction in childhood. He grew up the youngest of three in a family that was very dramatic and loud. Mom, the main dramatist, was verbally and physically abusive. She was also a committed pessimist, whose dire predictions permeated the household. Unfortunately, Cal's oldest brother was a superachiever; Cal could never do as well as his brother at anything. As a result, his mom directed a host of warnings his way. "*You will never pass exams. You are good for nothing. You will be sitting by the road with your begging bowl.*" As a result, he came into adulthood with several key beliefs: F*ailure means dire consequences. Something is wrong with me. I can't achieve success.* It's no wonder that he was stressed out all the time.

Cal's anxiety worsened when he went to university. He recalled being in the examination hall with his own abusive thoughts. "*I don't know this stuff. I'm going to fail. Mom is going to shout at me and label me. I can't do this.*" He also recognized how these thoughts had pursued him into his work life. From the beginning of his career, he constantly felt judged by his bosses and had this nagging feeling that he would never measure up. Like his mom, his first boss was a bully who said awful things to him. "*I don't know what you were thinking. I don't know where you will go from here. I don't see you growing with this company.*"

Callum started smoking as soon as he became a team leader heading up a major project at his company. In session, he clearly heard the defeatist thoughts running through his mind at the thought of this new responsibility. "*I am never going to succeed. I try so hard, but I will never reach the level I know I deserve.*" His anxiety skyrocketed immediately. Then that a colleague, who saw that he was stressing, handed him a cigarette so he could calm down. He was now a smoker.

Cal's turning point was being able to meet that younger part of himself in trance: the one who never felt good enough, who felt constantly judged, who never seemed to measure up to his older brother or his parent's expectations. He was able to tell his younger self, "*I am proud of you. I know you can achieve anything. I don't judge you. I totally and completely accept who you are.*" In effect, he became the kind, loving parent he never had for his own younger self. This key to self-acceptance and self-love was a game changer.

The second major shift occurred when Cal was able to vent out all the emotions he had held onto for decades - anger towards those bullies, fear of failure, anxiety, and stress were all released. Afterwards, he could finally accept that all he could do was his best - and that this was good enough. After he left my office, he never smoked again.

I ended up conducting sessions with Callum's son, too. At age 12, he began to get really anxious at exam time - to the point that he would have panic attacks and start to hyperventilate. As we worked through this, Callum realized that he had imprinted his same fear of failure and unrealistic expectations onto his son. "*I did this to him.*" Through hypnotherapy, we were finally able to break the chain for both father and son!

OUTCOME

Almost all smokers who can't quit for good will say something like, "*I was stressed out and I just I needed a cigarette.*" It's always stress that both leads them to relapse and to smoke in the first place. With these replacement smokers, cigarette takes on a persona. "It's always there for me," is what they often say. Not only are cigarettes a source of calm and clarity, to these smokers it represents unconditional friendship and support.

These smokers are completely unaware that cigarettes are attached to a deep void and emptiness within that seems unshakeable.

It wasn't until I incorporated hypnotherapy into my practice that I began to get the results I wanted with my smoking patients. When I heard a patient say, *"I have tried so many times to quit,"* I knew this was not just a physiological addiction, but an emotional one. These smokers not only crave the hit of dopamine; they crave their best friend - the one that helps them cope during times of stress and anxiety. With hypnotherapy, we can find the root of that anxiety and collapse all of the emotions underneath. Once we do this, we stop the desire to smoke dead in its tracks.

As a doctor, I tended to look at anxiety or stress as an entity unto itself. Yet with replacement smokers there is always a story behind the stress that is both unique and powerful.

"Stress is the symptom, not the cause."

Though all of these smokers had tough childhoods, they felt like they came through pretty intact. When I would initially ask them about their childhood, they wouldn't offer up any trauma or challenge. In fact, they would invariably say, "It was fine." But it was never fine. In every first session, the subconscious would automatically take my patient to the life experience that created that anxiety and the flow of emotions embedded in that childhood experience. As they put the pieces together, I could watch the lightbulb go on.

In the final session, I always ask smokers to bring their cigarettes and lighter with them. We have created new neural pathways that reinforce both their own inherent, positive coping mechanisms and the negative aspects of smoking. Then we get to test that out. At the end of this last session, I'll say, "*Now, smell your cigarettes.*" When they do, they are shocked to find they smell disgusting. This validates for them that those old neural pathways of addiction are no longer active.

Most of these patients get really worried that the desire to smoke will come back (because in the past, it always has). They need something that will give them a sense of control, so I teach them self-hypnosis. This is a powerful tool that both counteracts the withdrawal symptoms and allows them to deal with stress and anxiety in a new way. Self-hypnosis allows them to reinforce those positive neuropathways that we've established.

For any long-standing addiction, there is an embedded emotional program running that needs to be rewritten. Though I can't say it's easy - most addiction patterns require five back-to-back, very intense, sessions - the high success rate makes it totally worth it. With hypnotherapy, we challenge the power of that abusive, best friend relationship they have with their substance of choice - the "best friend" that actually steals their health and happiness - and we replace it with their own power.

CHAPTER SEVENTEEN

"We replace the void with love –
filling the emptiness that steals their health
and happiness with self-acceptance."

FREE RESOURCE

Are you a Replacement Smoker? Download this PDF questionnaire and find out.

https://www.enso-nia.com/within/resources

CHAPTER EIGHTEEN

THE VERSATILITY OF HYPNOTHERAPY IN MODERN MEDICINE

"We have barely scratched the surface."

One of the biggest reasons I chose to practice hypnotherapy full-time is the sheer excitement and creativity it has brought to my life. Hypnotherapy is not just for pain management, weight loss, or smoking cessation. Over the decades, hypnotherapy has evolved through contributions from the research and development in human mind sciences and clinical studies, as well as the influence of Eastern practices involving the mind. It has evolved from suggestive therapy to a profoundly transformative therapeutic intervention. This expansion of the breadth and scope of hypnotherapy allows us to deal with a vast array of health conditions and chronic ailments. I do wish to emphasize that the unbelievable breakthroughs in health and wellbeing that I have achieved in my work are no random occurrences. Firstly, I am sure that my medical background gives me a unique position to understand my client's conditions from a whole new perspective, compared to how a classical therapist would approach the very same condition.

Even more significantly, I was able to apply to full potential the knowledge of a technique called "Integrated Clinical Hypnotherapy." This is the method I have mastered. A significant upgrade to the classical hypnotherapy format, this is the knowledge that I now use to help transform my client's lives. I am equally passionate about teaching it to those who want to learn it.

The sheer versatility and consistency in addressing a diverse range of human conditions, as well as the breakthrough results and the quick turnaround times, have become a beacon of hope for so many who have struggled with mainstream medicine alone. This method has become the key catalyst for a silent revolution in the field of human health and wellbeing that opens up unlimited possibilities for modern medicine to make that paradigm shift.

I have had positive results with all forms of addiction, anxiety, phobias, depression, vertigo, and even infertility. The more sessions I undertake, the more I realize that I have barely scratched the surface of what hypnotherapy can do.

Through all the cases presented in this book, we have seen time and again that what the best of modern medical science failed to detect or resolve for a myriad of health issues, hypnotherapy was a critical factor in healing. It helped to unravel the underlying psychosomatic cause of health conditions that the best of laboratory equipment could not detect.

As such, I am convinced that hypnotherapy is a vital bridge which seamlessly connects modern medical practice to the core essence of the Human Mind Sciences. This connection instantly expands the scope of medicine and gives it a whole new dimension. It does this by taking into due consideration elements barely recognized by modern medicine, the very elements that define us as human beings - our thoughts, feelings, emotions, and their lasting impact on our physical health. This has been the greatest missing piece in mainstream medicine, specifically when it comes to chronic ailments. We now have a unique opportunity to revolutionize modern medicine. To make it complete. To make it whole.

To recognize the patient as a whole person, including the makeup of his thoughts, emotions, and their impact on the physical body - this integrated approach to healthcare will be the genesis of the practice of "Conscious Medicine," moving beyond a pharmacological or surgical approach.

The following thumbnail sketches illustrate even more ways in which hypnotherapy has been instrumental in uncovering the cause of conditions that would typically leave medical practitioners searching for answers. I hope these cases give you an even better idea of this creative, expansive, fluid therapy.

HABITS

"Whose attention am I seeking?"

It was my last consultation for the day. I heard a knock at my door, and a lean teenage girl dressed in a school uniform entered my room, accompanied by her mother. This girl, named Siri, seemed confident in her own way, though she had a sheepish smile on her face as she introduced herself. Upon asking what brings them to me, the mother pointed directly at Siri and said almost sarcastically: "Meet the 14-year-old who still sucks her thumb!" I sensed cynicism; however Siri appeared oblivious of her mother's tone...

Siri is a healthy 14-year-old with no previous medical history. She exhibited this tendency of thumb-sucking when she was a baby, stopped at the age of four or so, then suddenly began the behavior again at the age of seven. While it didn't necessarily bother Siri all that much – what was most peculiar was that she only sucked her thumb at home, so socially it wasn't an issue - her mother was at her wit's end. The moment Siri stepped foot in the house, her thumb went into her mouth. It was driving her mom absolutely mad.

Though it was mom who had the hardest time with it, it was Siri who found me, telling her mom, "*I want to see this doctor, I want to do hypnotherapy.*" Siri had actually researched hypnosis (and me!)

because she also felt something was amiss and wanted to get control over it.

In our only session together, I ask this teenager in trance to see that part of herself who is addicted to thumb-sucking. Immediately, she returns to a time when she is seven years old and her baby sister has been brought home from the hospital. Ah! In that moment something shifts and Siri in a blink understands her own behavior - this new baby has all of her parent's attention. Though she is happy to meet her baby sister, she is no longer the baby herself. Now she feels she has to grow up before she is ready. Sucking her thumb is a perfect way to *regain mom's attention*, as mom puts everything she has into getting Siri to stop.

In our session, my only intervention is to have teen Siri put her arms around her seven-year-old self, providing reassurance that she is seen and loved. Afterwards, I ask that seven-year-old to go to mom and put herself in her mom's arms. As the inner child settles into her mom, the older Siri tells me in awe, "*She's not sucking her thumb anymore!*"

The next day, I received the best text from Siri's mom. "I drove her back home [from your session] and she has not sucked her thumb at all. What did you do?"

PROPRIOCEPTION

"This problem is just ridiculous!"

Rija is a no-nonsense woman in her thirties who came to me with a very specific complaint of dizziness while driving on the highway; this, in turn, created a phobia of driving on highways. This had been going on for seven years, but she found a solution by avoiding routes with highways. Weirdly, this dizziness does not showcase in any other situation. That is, until six months before our session, when things changed after she moved to another country. Then she was forced to transport her son back and forth to school every day - and there was just no way to avoid highways. When she found me, she had been taking a cab (which wasn't sustainable). She realized this was illogical - *"This problem is just ridiculous!"* - but it was also very real, and she didn't know what to do.

Rija had already been to numerous physicians and had all the routine checkups, including several ENT exams. She was diagnosed with benign paroxysmal positional vertigo (BPPV) and prescribed various medications typical for this diagnosis, yet nothing seemed to work.

In our only session, I asked Rija to go back in time to the first instance when she experienced the dizzy sensation. She told me she was on the highway in her car and there was an accident. Traffic was all backed up. She felt dizzy, panicked, and had a feeling like she had to throw up. She wanted to pull over, but due to construction, there was no place to stop. "*There was no escape*."

My intervention here was simple. While in trance, I just had Rija do some easy breath work as a way to release that tension, anxiety, and panic. Still in trance, I did a double check that these energies were gone. I had her see herself back in her car, driving in the future on the exact highway she would need to take, to make sure the dizziness was completely gone. She reported that there was no more sensation. "*It is all clear*."

Rija wrote:

Dear Dr. Sonia,

Thank you so much. As you recollect, I had a severe phobia towards driving on highways and bridges. I can today happily say that my phobia and accompanying dizziness has gone away and I'm driving absolutely everywhere!

It has made my life so much easier and I drop my son off to school every day with complete ease and comfort. The hypnotherapy session also gave me a lot of positivity in all aspects of my daily life, which I hadn't realized I was lacking.

PHYSICAL RECOVERY

"I desire the best possible outcome."

Susan, a family physician with an interest in holistic wellness, was diagnosed with a 7x7 centimeter ovarian cyst. She had married two years before and wanted to start a family. Her inability to get pregnant led her to seek a fertility specialist who found the cyst.

Susan had put off surgery for as long as possible (several years, actually) because she knew the risks - lesions to one or both fallopian tubes and ovaries, bleeding, and infection. As a doctor, she also knew that post-op pain and nausea are almost inevitable, with a recovery period of a few weeks to a few months. None of this sounded particularly pleasant. Worse of all, complications could prevent her from becoming a mom.

Susan didn't come to me to heal the cyst, though. The endometrioma had become so large and painful that she had already scheduled it to be removed the following week. Her goal for hypnotherapy was to prepare for the best possible outcome for the surgery. As a holistic wellness geek, she knew the power of the mind.

During our first two meetings, we focused on clearing repressed emotions of guilt, shame, and self-criticism that Susan discovered in early childhood. She connected to this feeling of being deeply misunderstood as a kid, particularly by her family, who consistently labeled her as selfish. In reality, she was a spiritual child who always had the best intentions for others, but she was so filled with wonder and excitement that she could be a bit impulsive, assertive, and loud; she was just so happy and in awe of the world around her. Over time, she received the definitive message from those around her: Don't be so self-centered, dim your own light, and let your sister (who was quieter child) get some attention.

All of these emotions led to a black box of repressed energy that Susan visualized around her abdomen. As our work together released these energies, she was aware of positive emotions - strength, fortitude, self-acceptance, joy, wonder, freedom, and self-love - coming back to her. Interestingly, she felt these positive emotions returning to her abdomen as well, without any prompting from me.

In our final session, we also focused on creating a healthy reproductive system and the best possible outcome for Susan's surgery. In trance, I asked her to see the blueprint for a perfectly healthy reproductive system. As we began, her sense of her own reproductive functioning was at 33%, but as we ended, it was a 93%. We developed a very specific script of affirmations that the anesthesiologist would read as she was going under anesthetic. The script called for the surgery to proceed with ease, without damage to, or need to interfere with, her reproductive organs, minimal symptoms post-surgery, and a quick overall recovery.

In the end, the surgery went perfectly. Though it was four hours long, the entire cyst was removed, Susan's reproductive organs were intact, and her fallopian tubes were 100% patent. Her surgeon was amazed! The medical team couldn't believe that she has no nausea or vomiting post-surgery which is common after general anesthesia.

Susan describes her experience:

"When I woke up, I could not believe the procedure was done. The surgeon said the best possible outcome occurred; he removed the cyst without touching any reproductive organs! That week I took minimal pain medications, and I was up and walking the day after my procedure. My husband, who is also a physician, could not believe how good I looked the next day. He was convinced that hypnosis was a powerful tool! In my follow-up with the surgeon, he was surprised at how well I was recovering. He is also now a believer in the power of the mind to generate healing and positive surgical outcomes. I can't wait to share hypnosis with my patients to help them reach their own personal health and wellness goals."

CHAPTER NINETEEN

THE FUTURE IS OURS

"I don't talk limitations;
I talk possibilities."

Hypnotherapy once belonged to the world of medicine and I don't just believe - *I know* - that it's time to bring it back into mainstream use. It has the potential to improve outcomes, decrease suffering, mediate the usage of medication, boost overall health, and yes, even heal. And when we combine hypnotherapy tools such as "Integrated Clinical Hypnotherapy" with current medical treatment, I believe we can positively impact almost every disease state. We are on the cusp of a movement: one so powerful that it has the potential to revolutionize modern healthcare.

Many of us, my fellow physicians and patients alike, have been yearning to co-create this new kind of healthcare. I believe that, for some of you, the information in this book will bring clarity to see that matters of the mind and body are intimately connected. For others, this book will act as a catalyst. You will know who you are. Sheer curiosity combined with your desire to do more, go further, and make a bigger impact will pull you to take some kind of action within your field of influence.

Anyone can participate in this revolution. Whether you are overseeing the future of large healthcare conglomerates, or you are an individual practitioner serving your community. Whether you head a large educational institution grooming the next generation of mainstream medical students, or you lead the Integrative Medicine department's vision to integrate new and effective techniques. Whether you are focused on cutting-edge research on Mind-Body interventions, or just another person looking for nothing but hope, to relieve yourself from an age-old malady, and to enjoy life to its fullest. I see *all* of you as part of this movement.

My vision is to revolutionize our medical system. Through this amazing modality, I have both rediscovered the hopes I had as a young doctor and dared to redefine what is possible within my chosen field. It is my hope that I have inspired you to reach for something higher, too.

For those who want to join me on my journey, I dream of my fellow physicians becoming passionate advocates of the Mind-Body connection by getting trained in the mind science of hypnotherapy. I dream of offering the opportunity of this training to willing staff members in their clinics or organizations to upgrade their medical practice to a whole new level. I dream that all such consciously operating physicians will not just rely on refilling prescriptions, but will refer their patients with chronic diseases to hypnotherapy to address past experiences and emotions contributing to their illness.

"I dream that patients aren't seen by physicians as a disease label or a list of symptoms, but as a whole person with Body, Mind and Spirit."

I envision a medical system that freely explores new avenues, including different methods of research and scientific validation, to include the mind and emotions into the research mix.

"I dream of a medical system that feels expansive, fluid, collaborative, and dare I say, more human."

Let me now paint the grand vision I see in the very near future. It is a unique model of the future... with medical practitioners energized with a new zest for treating and healing and patients... experiencing never-before-seen improvements from chronic diseases without invasive treatments or prolonged dependency on chemicals.

It is something difficult to describe in words because it's almost overwhelming - but I know deep inside that this book is laying a foundation to that future reality! This vision has three distinct parts and each part is like a pillar giving this grand vision a solid foundation.

The first part of this grand vision involves showcasing everything I spoke of in the book as a practical workable model. I envision a medical facility dedicated to treating chronic illness in a brand-new way! A cutting-edge facility that combines advanced medical practices with the mind science of hypnotherapy in its most evolved form. This peaceful facility, filled with sunlight, white walls, plants, and a newfound awareness about "*Dis*-ease" will herald a new dawn of conscious medicine that, above all, will honor the mind as a powerful healing tool. As you enter this facility, each person who welcomes you has an ingrained understanding of the power of words. Anchored into the day-to-day operations of this facility is the core belief that all patients have the ability to heal themselves with targeted support from medical practitioners is.

At this facility I envision that, at the very first step when doctors take the medical history, they pause to ask about the patient's life experiences. Each patient's emotions are assessed and integrated into the treatment plan. All physicians here are trained in the use of the mind as a powerful healing tool, and through the department of Hypnotherapy (which does not exist in any medical facility currently) every patient is assigned to a hypnotherapist alongside their primary doctor. Patients receive the absolute best of Mind-Body medicine right there, as never before. A completely new paradigm!

Conscious prescription writing will be practiced as a standard protocol at this medical facility I envision, reducing and optimizing the use of medications. Every encounter is a marriage between physiology and the subconscious, a partnership between the physician and patient.

The second part of this grand vision is a deep desire to have this subject taught at medical schools so each medical student who becomes a future doctor has an in-depth understanding of the power of mind, and especially, the *power of words*! Each word we speak from the authority of being a medical professional carries a huge impact on our patients' minds. The fear unknowingly created when an unaware physician speaks of a disease can be detrimental; but it can just as easily be turned into hope through more supportive words if this awareness is ingrained from a very early stage at the medical school itself.

The third part of this grand vision is a cutting-edge research facility on Mind-Body medicine through all the cases being managed in this completely different way. We need to conduct more research encompassing various chronic ailments. This scientific data will help us move the world forward as more and more healthcare facilities become convinced to adopt this model.

Yes, this is a big vision – but in order to begin this enormous shift, physicians don't have to give up their medical practice like I did. There are so many ways to incorporate the amazing modality of *Integrated Clinical Hypnotherapy*, so get creative. Get trained yourself, or make training available to willing staff in your office. In fact, just start by asking your patients some probing questions and see what happens. I promise you that if find that your passion for what you do is waning, learning this modality will reawaken that spark. *There is so much we can do.*

A big vision takes big courage. In the end, this book is a call to be brave. It requires us to stop believing that small, incremental steps will get us to real change. But paradigm shifts that trigger movements and revolutions never come from playing it safe. This can feel scary, but taking even small steps can have a huge impact.

Will you join me in this movement? It's time. The future is ours to step into, together. Let's walk the path of wellness, hand in hand.

CHAPTER NINETEEN

BE BOLD. THE END RESULT IS WORTH IT!

ABOUT THE AUTHOR

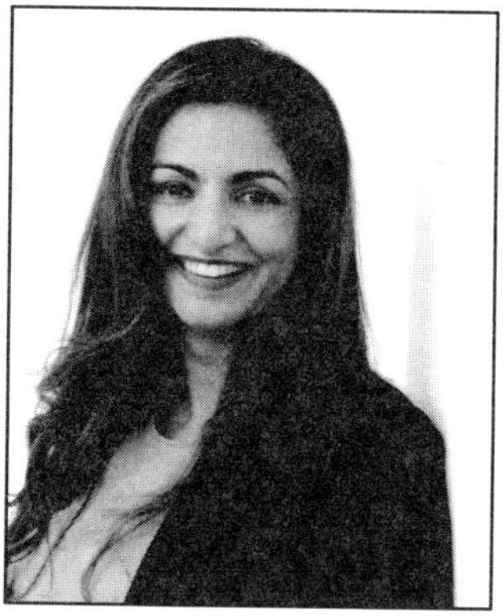

Dr. Sonia Gupte, CHt, is a family medicine physician, having practiced for 15 years in India, Singapore and Dubai. After discovering the power of the mind to transform the body, she relinquished her stethoscope and is now an internationally-known Board Certified Clinical Hypnotherapist and hypnotherapy trainer with clients in over 20 countries. She is the founder and director of Enso-nia Center for Mind and Life Transformation, an organization dedicated to revolutionizing the field of human wellness through the integration of hypnotherapy into mainstream healthcare. She has received her training from the internationally-renowned Dr. Brian Weiss as well as EKAA Foundation and TASSO Institute Holland. She lives in San Diego, California with her wonderful husband and two loving sons.

Connect with Dr. Gupte at:

www.enso-nia.com